DRUG CALCULATIONS
Process and Problems for Nursing Practice

DRUG CALCULATIONS
Process and Problems for Nursing Practice

Meta Brown, R.N. M.Ed.
Director, Division of Nursing,
Gateway Community College,
Phoenix, Arizona;
Chief Nurse,
403rd Combat Support Hospital,
Phoenix, Arizona

Joyce L. Mulholland, R.N.C., M.A., M.S.
Professor, Division of Nursing,
Gateway Community College,
Phoenix, Arizona

Third edition

The C. V. Mosby Company

St. Louis • Toronto • Washington, D.C.   1988

MOSBY

Editor: Nancy L. Coon
Developmental Editor: Susan R. Epstein
Production: Editing, Design & Production, Inc.
Book designer: Susan E. Lane

As new medical and nursing research and clinical experience broaden our knowledge, changes in treatment and drug therapy are required. The editors and the publisher of this work have made every effort to ensure that the drug dosage schedules herein are accurate and in accord with the standards accepted at the time of publication. Readers are advised, however, to check the product information sheet included in the package of each drug they plan to administer to be certain that changes have not been made in the recommended dose or in the contraindications for administration. This recommendation is of particular importance in regard to new or infrequently used drugs.

Third edition

The C.V. Mosby Company
11830 Westline Industrial Drive, St. Louis, Missouri 63146

Library of Congress Cataloging-in-Publication Data

Brown, Meta.
  Drug calculations.

  Rev. ed. of: Basic drug calculations. 2nd ed. 1984.
  Includes index.
  1. Pharmaceutical arithmetic—Problems, exercises, etc. I. Mulholland, Joyce L.
II. Brown, Meta. Basic drug calculations. [DNLM: 1. Drugs—administration & dosage—programmed instruction. QV 18 B879b]
RS57.B76 1988   615'.14   87-31396
ISBN 0-8016-0892-9

TT/VH/VH   9 8 7 6 5 4 3 2   03/D/374

Preface

The purpose of this workbook is to help health professionals understand the mathematics needed to calculate dosages for administration of medications. The book is easy to read and may be used as a self-instructional unit or with assistance from tutors or instructors. Each new concept is worked out in step-by-step examples. The solutions and proofs for problems are solved in detail in the answer section so students may verify each step of the process. The medication problems are clinically realistic and sequenced from simple to more difficult.

The book is divided into 12 chapters. Each chapter begins with objectives so students know exactly what to expect. A general mathematics pretest precedes Chapter 1. This diagnostic tool enables students to evaluate their foundation in mathematics before beginning the text and to determine the extent of their review needs and specific areas of weakness. The comprehensive examination that follows the last chapter provides an evaluative tool for the entire text.

This edition has been revised to include several visual aids that make learning easier. More problems have been added to each chapter, and the content has been updated to reflect current theory and clinical practice. The intravenous section has been divided into two chapters: ''Basic Intravenous Calculations'' and ''Intravenous Titrations.'' The expanded and reorganized material provides students with a thorough knowledge base in intravenous drug calculation and administration in a logical manner that proceeds from basic to advanced techniques.

Answers to all chapter problems, as well as the mathematics pretest and comprehensive examination, can be found at the end of the book. The perforated pages can be easily removed and placed next to the problems for comparison and review.

The ratio and proportion method is used throughout the text because, unlike other methods of calculation, it permits a logical, effective method of proving one's calculations. This enables students to check their own calculations as they learn and establishes the habit of verifying calculations. In view of the nurse's legal responsibility and accountability regarding administration of medication, this is a valuable habit to develop.

We thank Betty Gahart, R.N., author of *Intravenous Medications,* for allowing us to quote safe ranges of intravenous medications, and the publishers of the *Physicians' Desk Reference* for permission to quote medication dosage ranges.

Meta Brown

Joyce L. Mulholland

Contents

General mathematics pretest

Directions: Take this test completely. Then check your answers on page 135 to see which areas you may need to review.

Change to whole or mixed numbers:

1. $^{25}\!/_4$ 2. $^{36}\!/_7$

Change to improper fractions:

3. $4^2\!/_9$ 4. $9\frac{1}{2}$

Find the lowest common denominator (bottom number) in the following fractions:

5. $^4\!/_{11}$ and $\frac{1}{6}$ 6. $^2\!/_5$ and $^5\!/_9$

Add the following numbers:

7. $\frac{1}{5}$, $\frac{1}{6}$, and $^2\!/_3$ 8. $1\frac{1}{2} + 3\frac{1}{8} + 2\frac{1}{6}$

Subtract the following:

9. $^5\!/_7 - \frac{1}{4}$ 10. $8\frac{1}{4} - 3\frac{3}{8}$

Multiply the following:

11. $\frac{1}{6} \times \frac{1}{2}$ 12. $^2\!/_8 \times 1\frac{1}{3}$

Divide the following:

13. $\frac{1}{3} \div ^2\!/_5$ 14. $1\frac{1}{8} \div 2\frac{1}{2}$

Express the following fractions reduced to lowest terms (numbers):

15. $^3\!/_{150}$ 16. $^4\!/_{19}$

Write the following as decimals:

17. Fourteen hundredths   18. Three and sixteen thousandths

Add the following:

19. $3.04 + 1.865$ 20. $25.7 + 3.008$

Subtract the following:

21. $3 - 0.04$

22. $0.96 - 0.1359$

Multiply the following:

23. 0.003×1.2

24. 3×0.5

Divide the following and carry to the third decimal place:

25. $201.1 \div 20$

26. $20.6 \div 0.21$

Change the following to decimals:

27. $^{23}/_{43}$

28. $9\frac{1}{8}$

Solve the following percents:

29. 15% of 63

30. $1\frac{3}{4}$% of 4210

Change the following decimals to fractions:

31. 0.70

32. 0.492

33. Write 17% as a decimal and as a fraction.

34. Write $\frac{1}{8}$ as a decimal and as a percent.

35. Write 0.014 as a fraction and as a percent.

CHAPTER 1

General mathematics

Objectives

- Convert fractions into whole and mixed numbers.

- Change mixed numbers into improper fractions.

- Find lowest common denominators in fractions.

- Add fractions and mixed numbers and reduce to lowest terms (reduce fractions).

- Subtract fractions and mixed numbers.

- Multiply fractions and mixed numbers.

- Divide fractions and mixed numbers.

- Given two fractions, determine which is greater and which is smaller.

- Distinguish among decimal fractions in tenths, hundredths, ten-thousandths, and hundred-thousandths.

- Read whole numbers and decimal fractions.

- Divide decimals to third decimal place.

- Add, subtract, and divide decimals.

- Change decimals to fractions.

- Reduce fractions to lowest terms.

- Change fractions to decimals.

- Change percent to fraction.

- Convert fraction to decimal.

- Change percent to decimal.

- Convert decimal to percent.

- Find percent.

A fraction is part of a whole number. The fraction ⁶⁄₈ means that there are 8 parts to the whole number (bottom) but you want to measure only 6 of those parts (top number).

⁶⁄₈ can be reduced by division of both the numbers by 2.

$$\frac{6 \div 2}{8 \div 2} = \frac{3}{4}$$

Changing improper fractions into whole or mixed numbers

An improper fraction has a large numerator and a small denominator, such as ⁸⁄₄.

RULE:	**1** When the top number is larger than the bottom number, divide the bottom number into the top number.
	2 Write the remainder as a fraction and reduce to lowest terms.

EXAMPLE: ⁸⁄₄ = 8 ÷ 4 = 2   *Whole number*

¹⁶⁄₆ = 16 ÷ 6 = 2⁴⁄₆ = 2²⁄₃   *This is a mixed number* because it has a whole number plus a fraction.

[1A] **Worksheet**   (Answers on p. 136)

Change the following to whole numbers or mixed fractions:

1. ⁸⁄₈ =

2. ¹³⁄₄ =

3. ⁶⁄₂ =

4. ¹⁴⁄₉ =

5. ³⁴⁄₆ =

6. ¹⁰⁰⁄₂₅ =

7. ⁷⁄₄ =

8. ¹²⁰⁄₆₄ =

9. ¹²⁄₄ =

10. ⁴¹⁄₆ =

Changing mixed numbers into improper fractions

EXAMPLE: $2\frac{3}{8} = \dfrac{8 \times 2 + 3}{8} = \frac{19}{8}$

$4\frac{2}{5} = \dfrac{20 + 2}{5} = \frac{22}{5}$

1B Worksheet   (Answers on p. 136)

Change the following to improper fractions:

1. $1\frac{1}{5} =$ 5. $13\frac{3}{5} =$ 8. $2\frac{5}{8} =$

2. $1\frac{1}{4} =$ 6. $4\frac{3}{8} =$ 9. $10\frac{3}{6} =$

3. $16\frac{1}{3} =$ 7. $3\frac{5}{6} =$ 10. $125\frac{2}{3} =$

4. $3\frac{7}{12} =$

Addition of fractions and mixed numbers

Finding lowest common denominator (in fraction)

RULE: 1 Find the lowest common number that the bottom numbers can be divided into.
2 Change the fractions to equivalent fractions using these bottom numbers.

EXAMPLE: $\frac{2}{3} = \frac{16}{24}$
$\frac{7}{8} = \frac{21}{24}$
$\frac{1}{6} = \frac{4}{24}$

Addition of fractions and mixed numbers

RULE: 1 If fractions have the same bottom number, add the top numbers, write over the bottom number, and reduce.

EXAMPLE:
$$\begin{array}{r} \frac{1}{5} \\ +\frac{2}{5} \\ \hline \frac{3}{5} \end{array}$$

2 If fractions have different bottom numbers, find the lowest common number and then add the top numbers.

EXAMPLE:
$$\begin{array}{r} \frac{3}{5} \ = \ \frac{9}{15} \\ +\frac{2}{3} \ = \ +\frac{10}{15} \\ \hline \frac{19}{15} \ = 19 \div 15 = 1\frac{4}{15} \end{array}$$

3 To add mixed numbers, first add the fractions and then add this to the sum of the whole numbers.

EXAMPLE:
$$\begin{array}{r} 9\frac{5}{8} = \ 9\frac{15}{24} \\ +6\frac{1}{6} = \ \underline{6\ \frac{4}{24}} \\ 15\frac{19}{24} \end{array}$$

Worksheet (Answers on p. 136)

Add the following fractions and mixed numbers:

1. $\frac{1}{5}$
    $+\frac{2}{5}$

2. $\frac{3}{5}$
    $+\frac{2}{3}$

3. $6\frac{1}{6}$
    $+9\frac{5}{8}$

4. $1\frac{3}{8}$
    $+9\frac{9}{10}$

5. $2\frac{1}{4}$
    $+3\frac{1}{8}$

6. $\frac{1}{8}$
    $\frac{1}{4}$
    $+\frac{2}{9}$

7. $\frac{7}{9}$
    $\frac{4}{5}$
    $+\frac{9}{10}$

8. $3\frac{1}{4}$
    $+9\frac{3}{4}$

9. $8\frac{2}{5}$
    $14\frac{7}{10}$
    $+9\frac{9}{10}$

10. $2\frac{1}{3}$
    $4\frac{1}{6}$

Subtraction of fractions and mixed numbers

RULE: **1** If fractions have the same bottom number, find the difference between the top numbers and write it over the common number. Reduce the fraction if necessary.

EXAMPLE:

$$
\begin{array}{r}
^{27}\!/_{32} \\
-\,^{18}\!/_{32} \\
\hline
^{9}\!/_{32}
\end{array}
$$

Difference between the top numbers (27 minus 18) equals 9. Bottom number is 32.

RULE: **2** If fractions have different bottom numbers, find the lowest common bottom number and proceed as above.

EXAMPLE:

$$
\begin{array}{r}
^{7}\!/_{8} = \,^{21}\!/_{24} \\
-\,^{2}\!/_{3} = \,^{16}\!/_{24} \\
\hline
^{5}\!/_{24}
\end{array}
$$

Difference between the top numbers (21 minus 16) equals 5. Bottom number is 24.

RULE: **3** To subtract mixed numbers, first subtract the fractions and then find the difference in the whole numbers. If the fraction in the bottom number is larger than the fraction in the top number, you cannot subtract it. You must borrow from the whole number before subtracting the fraction.

EXAMPLE:

$$
\begin{array}{r}
21\,^{7}\!/_{16} \\
-\ 7\,^{12}\!/_{16}
\end{array}
$$

You cannot subtract the top numbers because 12 is larger than 7. Therefore, you must make a whole number out of $^{7}\!/_{16}$ and add the 7.

$$^{16}\!/_{16} + \,^{7}\!/_{16} = \,^{23}\!/_{16}$$

Because we added a whole number to the fraction, we must take a whole number away from 21 and make it 20. The problem now is set up as follows:

$$
21^{7}\!/_{16} = 20^{16}\!/_{16} + \,^{7}\!/_{16} =
\begin{array}{r}
20^{23}\!/_{16} \\
-\ 7^{12}\!/_{16} \\
\hline
13^{11}\!/_{16}
\end{array}
$$

RULE: **4** Reduce answer to lowest terms.

Worksheet   (Answers on p. 137)

Subtract fractions and mixed numbers (reduce answer to lowest terms):

1. $\frac{4}{5}$
    $-\frac{1}{2}$

2. $7\frac{16}{24}$
    $-3\frac{1}{8}$

3. $21\frac{7}{16}$
    $-\ 7\frac{12}{16}$

4. $\frac{27}{32}$
    $-\frac{18}{32}$

5. $6\frac{3}{10}$
    $-2\frac{1}{5}$

6. $\frac{7}{8}$
    $-\frac{2}{3}$

7. $3\frac{5}{8}$
    $-1\frac{3}{8}$

8. $5\frac{3}{7}$
    $-1\frac{6}{7}$

9. 7
    $-1\frac{3}{4}$

10. $2\frac{7}{8}$
    $-\ \frac{3}{4}$

Multiplication of fractions and mixed numbers

RULE:
1 Change mixed number to improper fraction.
2 Cancel if possible by dividing any top and bottom number by the largest number contained in each.
3 Multiply remaining top number to find top-number result.
4 Multiply bottom number to find bottom-number result.
5 Reduce answer to lowest terms.

EXAMPLE:

$$1 \quad \tfrac{4}{5} \times {}^{15}\!/_{16} = \frac{\overset{1}{\cancel{4}}}{\cancel{5}} \times \frac{\overset{3}{\cancel{15}}}{\cancel{16}} = \tfrac{3}{4}$$

$$2 \quad 4\tfrac{1}{2} \times 2\tfrac{1}{4} = \frac{9}{2} \times \frac{9}{4} = \frac{81}{8} = 10\tfrac{1}{8}$$

$$3 \quad 6 \times \tfrac{3}{8} = \frac{6}{1} \times \frac{3}{8} = \frac{\overset{3}{\cancel{6}}}{1} \times \frac{3}{\underset{4}{\cancel{8}}} = \frac{9}{4} = 2\tfrac{1}{4}$$

| 1E | **Worksheet** (Answers on p. 138) |

Multiply the following fractions and mixed numbers (reduce answer to lowest terms):

1. $\tfrac{1}{3} \times \tfrac{2}{4} =$

2. $5\tfrac{1}{2} \times 3\tfrac{1}{8} =$

3. $1\tfrac{3}{4} \times 3\tfrac{1}{7} =$

4. $4 \times 3\tfrac{1}{8} =$

5. $\tfrac{2}{4} \times 2\tfrac{1}{6} =$

6. $\tfrac{1}{5} \times \tfrac{1}{3} =$

7. $\tfrac{3}{4} \times \tfrac{5}{8} =$

8. $\tfrac{5}{6} \times 1\tfrac{9}{16} =$

9. $\tfrac{5}{100} \times 900 =$

10. $2\tfrac{1}{10} \times 4\tfrac{1}{3} =$

■ 10

Division of fractions and mixed numbers

> **RULE:**
> **1** Change mixed number to improper fractions.
> **2** Turn the number after the ÷ (division) sign upside down.
> **3** Follow steps for multiplying and reduce any fractions.

EXAMPLE: **1** $\dfrac{1}{2} \div \dfrac{5}{8} = \dfrac{1}{2} \times \dfrac{8}{5} = \dfrac{8}{10} = \dfrac{4}{5}$

$$\textbf{2}\ \ 8\tfrac{3}{4} \div 15 = \dfrac{35}{4} \times \dfrac{1}{15} = \dfrac{\overset{7}{\cancel{35}}}{4} \times \dfrac{1}{\underset{3}{\cancel{15}}} = \dfrac{7}{12}$$

1F **Worksheet**   (Answers on p. 138)

Divide the following fractions and mixed numbers:

1. $\frac{2}{5} \div \frac{5}{8} =$ 6. $\frac{3}{4} \div 6 =$

2. $8\frac{3}{4} \div 15 =$ 7. $2 \div \frac{1}{5} =$

3. $\frac{3}{4} \div \frac{1}{8} =$ 8. $3\frac{3}{8} \div 4\frac{1}{2} =$

4. $\frac{1}{16} \div \frac{1}{4} =$ 9. $\frac{3}{5} \div \frac{3}{8} =$

5. $\frac{1}{3} \div \frac{1}{2} =$ 10. $4 \div 2\frac{1}{8} =$

Value of fractions

RULE: The smaller the bottom number of a fraction, the greater it is in value. Make a whole number out of a fraction to see which one is larger.

EXAMPLE: ⅙ is greater than ⅑ because the bottom number is smaller.

RULE: To make a whole number out of the fraction ⁶⁄₆ means there are 6 parts to the whole number.

EXAMPLE: $\frac{1}{6}$ $\frac{1}{6}$ $\frac{1}{6}$ $\frac{1}{6}$ $\frac{1}{6}$ $\frac{1}{6}$ = 6 parts   Each ⅙ part is larger than the ⅑ part.

$\frac{1}{9}$ $\frac{1}{9}$ $\frac{1}{9}$ $\frac{1}{9}$ $\frac{1}{9}$ $\frac{1}{9}$ $\frac{1}{9}$ $\frac{1}{9}$ $\frac{1}{9}$ = 9 parts   Each ⅑ part is smaller than the ⅙ part.

Which would you rather have: $\frac{1}{6}$ or $\frac{1}{9}$ of your favorite pie?

1G Worksheet (Answers on p. 139)

Solve the following problems:

1. Which is greater: ⅓ or ⅕?

2. Which is smaller: ¹⁄₁₀₀ or ¹⁄₁₅₀?

3. Which is greater: ¹⁄₂₅₀ or ¹⁄₃₀₀?

4. Which is smaller: ⅙ or ⅛?

In the following problems, *estimate* answers before beginning. This is a good habit to develop.

5. Doctor ordered gr $\frac{1}{150}$. On hand you have gr $\frac{1}{200}$ tablets. Will you need to give more or less than what is on hand?

6. On hand you have gr $\frac{1}{150}$ tablets. Doctor ordered gr $\frac{1}{300}$. Will you need to give more or less than what is on hand?

7. Doctor ordered gr $\frac{1}{6}$. You have on hand gr $\frac{1}{4}$ tablets. Will you need more or less than what is on hand?

8. Doctor ordered gr $\frac{1}{10}$. On hand you have gr $\frac{1}{4}$ tablets. Will you need to give more or less than what is on hand?

9. On hand you have gr $\frac{1}{200}$. Doctor ordered gr $\frac{1}{100}$. Will you need to give more or less than what is on hand?

10. Doctor ordered gr $\frac{1}{8}$. On hand you have gr $\frac{1}{6}$ tablets. Will you need to give more or less than what is on hand?

Value of decimals

A decimal fraction is a fraction whose denominator (bottom number) is 10, 100, 1000, 10,000, and so on. It differs from a common fraction in that the denominator (bottom number) is *not* written but is expressed by the proper placement of the decimal point.

Observe the scale below. All whole numbers are to the left of the decimal point; all decimal fractions are to the right.

RULE:	**1** All whole numbers are to the left of the decimal; all decimal fractions are to the right of the decimal point.
	2 To read a decimal fraction, read the number to the right of the decimal and use the name that applies to "place value" of the *last* figure. All decimal fractions read with a *ths* on the end, except *half* and *thirds*.

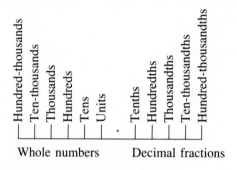

EXAMPLE: 0.257 = Two-hundred-fifty-seven thousand*ths*
0.2057 = Two-thousand-fifty-seven ten-thousand*ths*
0.20057 = Twenty-thousand-fifty-seven hundred-thousand*ths*

RULE:	**3** To read a whole number and a fraction, the decimal point reads as an *and*.

EXAMPLE: 327.006 = Three hundred twenty-seven *and* six thousand*ths*

Read the following out loud:

1. 0.08   3. 0.0017   5. 0.0006

2. 0.092   4. 3287.467   6. 100.01

Express the following as decimal fractions:

7. Thirty-six hundredths   _____

8. Three thousandths   _____

9. Eight ten-thousandths   _____

10. Two and seventeen thousandths   _____

11. Five hundredths   _____

12. Four and one tenth   _____

13. Twenty-four and two tenths   _____

14. Fifteen and one hundredth   _____

15. Nine and two ten-thousandths   _____

16. Three and eight thousandths   _____

17. One hundred and eighteen thousandths _____

18. Eighteen and fifteen hundredths   _____

19. Fifty-five thousandths   _____

20. Thirty-four and one tenth   _____

Division of decimals

EXAMPLE: $15 \div 6.2 = 6.2 \overline{)15.0.000}$

$$
\begin{array}{r}
2.419 \\
6.2\,\overline{)15.0.000} \\
12\ 4 \\ \hline
2\ 6\ 0 \\
2\ 4\ 8 \\ \hline
1\ 20 \\
62 \\ \hline
580 \\
558 \\ \hline
22
\end{array}
$$

Worksheet (Answers on p. 140)

Divide the following and carry to the *third* decimal place if necessary:

1. 158.4 ÷ 48

6. 78.6 ÷ 2.43

2. 200 ÷ 6.0

7. 26.78 ÷ 8.2

3. 15.06 ÷ 6

8. 266.5 ÷ 5.78

4. 79.4 ÷ 0.87

9. 10.80 ÷ 6.5

5. 670.8 ÷ 0.78

10. 76.53 ÷ 10

Addition of decimals

EXAMPLE: 0.8   3.27
          +0.5   +0.06
           1.3   3.33

REMEMBER: Line up the decimal points.

| 1J | **Worksheet**   (Answers on p. 141)

Add the following decimals:

1. $0.8 + 0.5 =$

2. $3.27 + 0.06 + 2 =$

3. $5.01 + 2.999 =$

4. $15.6 + 0.19 + 200 =$

5. $210.79 + 2 + 68.4 =$

6. $88.6 + 576.46 + 79.0 =$

7. $6.77 + 102 + 88.3 =$

8. $79.4 + 68.44 + 3.00 =$

9. $10.56 + 356.4 =$

10. $99.7 + 293.23 =$

Multiplication of decimals

RULE: **1** Multiply as in multiplying whole numbers.
2 Find the total number of decimal places in the multiplier *and* in the number to be multiplied.
3 Start from the right and count off the same number of places in the answer.
4 If the answer does not have enough places, supply as many zeros as needed.

EXAMPLE: $2.6 \times 0.0002 =$ 2.6 (1 decimal place)
$\underline{\times 0.0002}$ (4 decimal places)
0.00052 (5 decimal places starting at the right in the answer)

1K **Worksheet**   (Answers on p. 141)

Multiply the following decimals:

1. $3.14 \times 0.002 =$

2. $95.26 \times 1.125 =$

3. $100 \times 0.5 =$

4. $2.14 \times 0.03 =$

5. $36.8 \times 70.1 =$

6. $203.7 \times 28 =$

7. $88 \times 90.1 =$

8. $2.76 \times 0.003 =$

9. $54.5 \times 21 =$

10. $200 \times 0.2 =$

Subtraction of decimals

RULE: **1** Write decimals in a column, keeping the decimal points under each other.
2 Subtract as in whole numbers.
3 Place the decimal point in the answer directly under the decimal point in the sums to be added (zeros can be added *after* the decimal point without changing the value).

EXAMPLE: $0.6 - 0.524 = $ 0.600
                              -0.524
                              0.076
REMEMBER: Line up the decimal points.

1L **Worksheet**   (Answers on p. 142)

Subtract the following decimals:

1. $98.4 - 66.50 =$

2. $108.56 - 5.40 =$

3. $0.450 - 0.367 =$

4. $21.78 - 19.88 =$

5. $266.44 - 0.56 =$

6. $7.066 - 0.200 =$

7. $34.678 - 0.502 =$

8. $78.567 - 6.77 =$

9. $1.723 - 0.683 =$

10. $0.8100 - 0.6701 =$

Changing decimals to fractions

EXAMPLE:

1 0.375 has 3 numbers to the *right* of the decimal. To make a fraction out of 0.375 and also get rid of the decimal, just put it over 1000.

0.375 written as a fraction is $375/1000$.

It's easy to remember: 3 numbers on top and 3 zeros on the bottom.

2 0.90 written as a fraction is $90/100$.

The idea is the same as above: 2 numbers on top and 2 zeros on the bottom.

Worksheet (Answers on p. 142)

Work problems and reduce to lowest terms:

1. 0.40 =   6. 0.500 =

2. 0.8 =   7. 0.750 =

3. 0.250 =   8. 0.20 =

4. 4.08 =   9. 0.65 =

5. 1.32 =   10. 0.700 =

Changing common fractions to decimals

RULE:	**1** Divide the top number by the bottom number and place the decimal point in the proper position.

$$
\text{EXAMPLE:} \quad \frac{2}{5} = 5\overline{)2.00} \quad \begin{array}{c} 0.40 = 0.4 \\ \underline{2.0} \\ 0 \end{array}
$$

1N **Worksheet**   (Answers on p. 143)

Carry out division to *third* decimal place:

1. $^{19}/_{100} =$

2. $^9/_7 =$

3. $5^9/_{16} =$

4. $^1/_5 =$

5. $^2/_3 =$

6. $^1/_2 =$

7. $^1/_{12} =$

8. $^6/_8 =$

9. $^{15}/_{200} =$

10. $^{20}/_8 =$

Percentages, decimals, and fractions

The term *percent* and its symbol (%) mean hundred*ths*. A percent number is a fraction whose top number is already known and whose bottom is *always* understood to be 100.

Changing a percent to a fraction

RULE: The top number is the percent and the bottom number is always 100.

EXAMPLE: **1** 5% written as a fraction is $5/100$.

Drop the percent sign when converting 5% to $5/100$.

2 $1/2$% is written as a fraction $\dfrac{1/2}{100}$. You cannot leave the problem like this. $\dfrac{1/2}{100}$ means $1/2 \div 100 = 1/2 \times 1/100 = 1/200$. The problem is completed when $\dfrac{1/2}{100} = 1/2 \times 1/100 = 1/200$.

Converting a fraction to a decimal

RULE: **1** The fraction $5/100$ can be made into a decimal by dividing the bottom number into the top number.

EXAMPLE: **1** To change $5/100$ into a decimal means $5 \div 100$.

$$100\overline{)\begin{array}{l}.05 \\ 5.00 \\ \underline{5\ 00}\end{array}}$$ Don't forget the decimal point.

2 Change $1/200$ to a decimal. Divide the bottom number into the top number.

$$1 \div 200 = 200\overline{)\begin{array}{l}.005 \\ 1.000 \\ \underline{1\ 000}\end{array}}$$

Changing a percent to a decimal

RULE:	**1** A percent number can be changed to a decimal by having its decimal point moved 2 places to the *left* to signify hundred*ths*.

EXAMPLE: **1** 5% written as a decimal is 0.05.

REMEMBER: Move the decimal 2 places to the *left* and drop the % sign.

2 0.5% written as a decimal is 0.005.

REMEMBER: Move the decimal 2 places to the *left* and drop the % sign.

Converting a decimal to a percent

RULE:	**1** The only thing you must do is to move the decimal point 2 places to the *right* and add the percent sign.

EXAMPLE: **1** 0.05 is a decimal. To make it a percent, move the decimal point 2 places to the *right* and add the % sign. Therefore 0.05 = 5%.

2 0.005 = 0.5% or ½%

10 Worksheet   (Answers on p. 144)

	Fraction	Decimal	Percent
1.	_____	_____	66⅔%
2.	½	_____	_____
3.	_____	_____	6.5%
4.	¹⁄₁₂	_____	_____
5.	³⁄₁₀₀₀	_____	_____
6.	_____	0.10	_____
7.	_____	_____	250%
8.	_____	0.35	_____
9.	⅘	_____	_____
10.	_____	_____	78%

If you are having difficulty with fractions, decimals, or percents, review pp. 24–25 or see your instructor.

Finding the percentage

EXAMPLE: 23% of 64 = 64 × 0.23 = 14.72

| 1P | **Worksheet**   (Answers on p. 144) |

1. 114% of 240 =

2. 2% of 1500 =

3. ½% of 9328 =

4. ⅓% of 930 =

5. 28% of 50 =

6. 9% of 200 =

7. 120% of 400 =

8. 5% of 105.80 =

9. 10% of 520 =

10. 3% of 40.80 =

■ General Mathematics Test   (Answers on p. 145)

Change to whole or mixed numbers:

1. $^{34}/_6$ 2. $^{48}/_7$

Change to improper fractions:

3. $13^3/_5$ 4. $3^5/_6$

Find the lowest common bottom number in the following fractions:

5. $^{17}/_{20}$ and $^4/_5$ 6. $^7/_8$ and $^3/_5$

Add the following numbers:

7. $^1/_{18}$, $^1/_4$, and $^2/_9$ 8. $5^1/_8$, $1^1/_4$, and $4^1/_2$

Subtract the following:

9. $^7/_8 - ^2/_3$ 10. $6^2/_4 - 5^1/_2$

Multiply the following:

11. $^1/_5 \times ^1/_3$ 12. $^5/_6 \times ^2/_8$

Divide the following:

13. $^3/_4 \div ^1/_8$ 14. $3^3/_8 \div 4^1/_2$

Express the following ratios as fractions reduced to lowest terms (numbers):

15. 2:500   16. 2:13

Write the following as decimals:

17. Thirty-six hundredths _____   18. Two and seventeen thousandths _____

Add the following:

19. 5.01 + 2.999

20. 36.87 + 8.26 + 15.84

Subtract the following:

21. 4 − 0.176

22. 0.41 − 0.2538

Multiply the following:

23. 0.0005 × 0.02

24. 5 × 0.7

Divide the following and carry to the third decimal place:

25. 158.4 ÷ 48

26. 79.4 ÷ 0.87

Change the following to decimals:

27. $^{57}/_{48}$

28. 8$^{1}/_{16}$

Solve the following percents:

29. 24% of 52

30. 6¼% of 9328

Change the following decimals to fractions:

31. 0.400

32. 0.285

33. Write 43% as a decimal and as a fraction.

34. Write ¹/₁₀ as a decimal and as a percent.

35. Write 0.029 as a fraction and as a percent.

CHAPTER 2

Ratio and proportion

Objectives

- *Express ratios as fractions.*
- *Reduce fractions to lowest numerical terms.*
- *Solve ratio/proportion problems for x.*
- *Solve verbal and numerical ratio/proportion problems for x.*
- *Solve one-step ratio/proportion problems.*
- *Estimate answers.*
- *Prove answers.*

Ratio

> **RULE:** A ratio indicates the relationship of one quantity to another. It indicates *division* and may be expressed in fraction form.

EXAMPLE: $\frac{1}{3}$ may be expressed as a ratio 1:3.

2A **Worksheet** (Answers on p. 145)

Express the following ratios as fractions reduced to lowest terms:

1. 2:4	5. 43:86	8. 1:5
2. 4:6	6. 2:13	9. 1:150
3. 2:500	7. 7:49	10. 4:100
4. 6:1000		

Proportion

A proportion shows the relationship between two equal ratios. A proportion may be expressed as $3:5::6:10$ or $3:5 = 6:10$.

To solve the ratio and proportion problems, just do this:

RULE:
1 Multiply the two inside numbers.
2 Multiply the two outside numbers.
3 The answers should be the same.

EXAMPLE:

$3:5::6:10$

multiply

multiply

Multiply the two *inside* numbers: $5 \times 6 = 30$
Multiply the two *outside* numbers: $3 \times 10 = 30$

How to solve the problem when one of the numbers is unknown or x

Multiply the x first and put it on the *left* side of the equation.

EXAMPLE:

$3:5::x:10$

Multiply inside numbers: $5x$. Multiply outside numbers: $3 \times 10 = 30$. The equation will now look like this: $5x = 30$.

4 Now you must get x to stand alone. Cancel it out, and you will never go wrong. Whatever you do to one side you must do to the other to keep them equal. Canceling out eliminates the chance of dividing the wrong sides into each other. The end product of canceling out is a fraction, that is $^{30}/_5$.

A fraction means that the bottom number is always divided into the top number.

EXAMPLE: This cancels the 5 out: $\dfrac{\cancel{5}x}{\cancel{5}} = \dfrac{30}{5}$

5 The only part of the problem left unsolved is $^{30}/_5$. As you know, $^{30}/_5$ means $30 \div 5 = 6$; so $x = 6$.

Put the entire problem together, following the five steps outlined above. Remember to always put x on the *left*-hand side.

multiply

$3:5::x:10$ or $\begin{smallmatrix} 3 \\ 5 \end{smallmatrix} \times \begin{smallmatrix} x \\ 10 \end{smallmatrix}$

multiply

$5x = 30$ $5x = 30$

What you do to one side of the equation you must do to the other. This cancels out the 5 and leaves x.

$$\frac{\cancel{5}x}{\cancel{5}} = \frac{30}{5} \qquad \text{This means } 30 \div 5 \text{ or } 5\overline{)30}$$

$$x = 6 \qquad\qquad\qquad \frac{30}{0}$$

How do you know your answer is correct?

To *prove* your answer, just substitute the answer for the x in the problem, multiply the inside numbers together, and then multiply the outside numbers together.

EXAMPLE: PROOF: $3:5::6:10$

$$5 \times 6 = 30$$
$$3 \times 10 = 30$$

Now you are ready to solve for x.

2B Worksheet (Answers on p. 145)

Solve the following problems for x:

1. $\frac{1}{2}:x::1:8$

2. $9:x::5:300$

3. $\frac{1}{1000}:\frac{1}{100}::x:60$

4. $\frac{1}{4}:500::x:1000$

5. $36:12::\frac{1}{100}:x$

6. $6:24::0.75:x$

7. $x:600::4:120$

8. $0.7:70::x:1000$

9. $9:27::300:x$

10. $6:12::\frac{1}{4}:x$

Worksheet   (Answers on p. 147)

REMEMBER: Multiply two inside numbers, multiply two outside numbers, put x on the *left*.

Solve for x:

1. $\frac{1}{200}:x::1:800$

2. $15:30::x:12$

3. $\frac{1}{1000}:\frac{1}{100}::x:30$

4. $6:12::0.25:x$

5. $300:5::x:\frac{1}{60}$

6. $\frac{1}{150}:\frac{1}{200}::2:x$

7. $\frac{1}{2}:\frac{1}{6}::\frac{1}{4}:x$

8. $7.5:12::x:28$

9. $15:x::1.5:10$

10. $10:x::0.4:12$

Ratio and proportion: how to set up

> **RULE:**   **1** To set up a ratio and proportion, you must always put on the *left*-hand side what you already *have* or what you already *know*.
>
> **2** On the *right*-hand side you will put your x or what you *want* to know.
>
> **3** Each side of the equation is set up the *same way*.

EXAMPLE: Apples:*Pears*::Apples:x *Pears*

RULE:	**4** Multiply the two inside numbers. Multiply the two outside numbers.
	5 Always put *x* on the *left*.
	6 Prove all answers and label.

EXAMPLE: You wish to make a floral bouquet of 6 daffodils for every 4 roses. How many daffodils will you use for 30 roses?

Know   **Want to know**

6 daffodils:4 roses::*x* daffodils:30 roses   PROOF: $4 \times 45 = 180$

$$\frac{4x}{4} = \frac{180}{4} = 180 \div 4 = 45 \qquad\qquad 6 \times 30 = 180$$

Left

$4x = 180$

$x = 45$ daffodils

2D | **Worksheet**   (Answers on p. 149)

Problems to set up and prove:

1. You have a recipe for cocoa—4 scoops make 6 cups of cocoa. You want to make 18 cups for a party. How many scoops of cocoa? Set up a proportion.

2. You are making coffee, and 7 scoops make 8 cups. How many scoops make 40 cups?

3. You have to make a fruit basket with 6 bananas for every 9 apples. How many bananas for 72 apples?

4. Doctor ordered 450 mg of aspirin. On hand you have 300 mg in 1 tablet. How many tablets will you give?

5. You wish to plant 8 bushes for every 2 trees in your yard. How many bushes for 36 trees? (Estimate and prove.)

6. Doctor ordered 4 cups of All-Bran every day. How many days would it take to consume 84 cups of All-Bran? (Estimate and prove.)

7. It takes 4 cups of flour to make 3 loaves of bread. How many loaves of bread can be made from 24 cups of flour?

8. Your recipe for punch calls for 3 cups of soda for every ½ cup of fruit juice. How many cups of soda will you need for 2 cups of fruit juice?

9. You need 4 tbsp of sugar for every glass of lemonade you prepare. How many tablespoons of sugar will you need for 6 glasses of lemonade?

10. Doctor ordered 4 capsules every day. How many capsules would you need for 14 days?

Ratio and proportion: how to set up

> **RULE:**
>
> **1** You already know that what you *have* or what you know goes on the *left*-hand side of the equation. What you want to know goes on the *right*-hand side; so this will be the side for the *x*, or unknown.
>
> **2** Remember that both sides of the equation *must* be set up the same way.

EXAMPLE: Make a necklace that has 19 blue beads for every 1 yellow bead. How many blue beads are needed if you have 8 yellow beads?
(Prove your answer.)

Have   **Want to know**

19 blue beads:1 yellow bead::*x* blue beads:8 yellow beads

——— multiply ———
——— multiply ———

$1x = 152$ blue beads needed   PROOF: $19 \times 8 = 152$
                                                  $1 \times 152 = 152$

2E Worksheet   (Answers on p. 151)

Work problems and prove:

1. Doctor ordered 40 mg of aspirin. You have on hand 5 mg tablets. How many tablets will you give? Prove your answer and label.

2. Ordered is ¼ gr of codeine. You have on hand ⅙ gr tablets. **a,** Will you give *more* or *less* than what you have on hand? **b,** Set up proportion and prove.

3. Doctor ordered ⅙ gr of morphine. You have on hand ⅛ gr in 1 tablet. **a,** Will you give *more* or *less* of what you have? **b,** Do your work and prove.

4. The doctor tells you to drink 3 glasses of H_2O and eat 2 apples every day. How many apples will you have eaten when you have drunk 24 glasses of water?

5. If you were going to give all the teachers 6 pens for every 8 pencils, how many pens would you give for 72 pencils?

6. If you were making an omelet with ½ tsp of salt for every 3 eggs, how much salt would you use for 30 eggs?

7. If your coffeemaker makes 8 cups of coffee for every 7 scoops of coffee, how many scoops would you need to make 24 cups of coffee?

8. Your flower arrangements call for 5 carnations for each fern. How many carnations would you need to order for 10 ferns?

9. If you need 2 tbsp of vinegar for each cup of water, how many tablespoons would you need for 10 cups of water?

10. Ordered is 500 mg of Lincocin. You have on hand 250 mg per capsule. Will you give *more* or *less* of what you have? Set up proportion and prove.

■ Ratio and Proportion Test (Answers on p. 153)

SHOW ALL WORK.

Solve the following proportions for x:

1. $9:x::5:300$

2. $6:24::0.75:x$

3. $8:16::x:24$

4. $x:600::4:120$

5. $5:3000::15:x$

6. $0.7:70::x:1000$

7. $9:27::300:x$

8. $6:12::\frac{1}{4}:x$

9. $25:x::75:3000$

10. $0.6:10::0.5:x$

CHAPTER 3

Metric system

Objectives

- *Convert milligrams, grams, and kilograms.*

- *Memorize milliliter and liter conversions.*

- *Calculate gram and milligram conversion problems.*

- *Calculate one-step metric conversion problems by ratio and proportion method.*

- *Identify one- and two-step metric conversion problems.*

- *Calculate two-step metric conversion problems by ratio and proportion method.*

Explanation

The metric system is now being used exclusively in the *United States Pharmacopeia* and before long will probably be the only system used in drug dosage. Arabic numbers and decimals are used with this system. Blame the French if you don't like the metric system, but it's really easier than any other method because it is a decimal system (based on the number 10) and all the math involved is done by moving decimals.

The basic metric units are multiplied and divided always by a multiple of 10 to form the entire system. (The period for abbreviation often may not appear in some writings.) There are only a few equivalents that are used in medicine. These are as follows:

MEMORIZE:

Weight

1 mg (milligram)	= 1000 μg (or mcg) (micrograms)
1 g (gram)	= 1000 mg (milligrams)
1 kg (kilogram) = 2.2 lb	= 1000 g or Gm (grams)

Volume

1000 ml (milliliters) or cc (cubic centimeters) = 1 L (liter)

A milliliter (ml) is equivalent to a cubic centimeter (cc), and for all practical purposes these units may be used interchangeably. However, the use of milliliter is preferable. Hence:

$$1000 \text{ cc} = 1 \text{ L (liter)}$$
$$1000 \text{ ml} = 1 \text{ L (liter)}$$

PLEASE NOTE: The symbol, such as g or mg, always *follows* the amount.

EXAMPLE: 1000 mg
            1 g

■ Metric measurements, prefixes, and their equivalents

Prefix	Numerical value	Power of base 10	Meaning
giga	1,000,000,000.	10^9	One billion times
mega	1,000,000.	10^6	One million times
*kilo	1,000.	10^3	One thousand times
hecto	100.	10^2	One hundred times
deka	10.	10^1	Ten times
deci	.1	10^{-1}	Tenth part of
*centi	.01	10^{-2}	Hundredth part of
*milli	.001	10^{-3}	Thousandth part of
*micro	.000001	10^{-6}	Millionth part of
*nano	.000000001	10^{-9}	Billionth part of

These prefixes can be combined with liters and grams.

*Prefixes most frequently used in computing dosages.

	Weight	Volume
EXAMPLE:	decigram (dg)	deciliter (dl)
	dekagram (dkg)	dekaliter (dkl)
	hectogram (hg)	hectaliter (hl)
	centigram (cg)	centiliter (cl)
	kilogram (kg)	kiloliter (kl)
	milligram (mg)	milliliter (ml)

NOTE: Some doctors may use the symbol mgm for mg (milligram) and Gm for g (gram). The symbol mcg is becoming obsolete.

Conversions

1 g = 1000 mg

RULE:	The metric system is a decimal system. To convert g (large) to mg (small), multiply by 1000 or move the decimal point 3 places to the right (for *1000* times smaller). To convert mg (small) to g (large), divide by *1000* or move the decimal point 3 places to the left (for *1000* times greater).

EXAMPLE: We know 1000 mg = 1 g.
1500 mg = 1.5 g.
Divide 1500 mg by 1000 × 1.5 g, or move decimal 3 places to the left for converting mg (small) to g (large).
5 g = 5000 mg.
Multiply 5 g by 1000 = 5000 mg, or move decimal 3 places to the right for converting g (large) to mg (small).

3A Worksheet   (Answers on p. 154)

REMEMBER: 1 g = 1000 mg

1. 1 g = _____ mg

2. 2 g = _____ mg

3. 1.5 g = _____ mg

4. 0.5 g = _____ mg

5. ½ g = _____ mg

6. 0.25 g = _____ mg

7. 0.05 g = _____ mg

8. 0.1 g = _____ mg

9. 1.1 g = _____ mg

10. 0.3 g = _____ mg

11. 25 mg = _____ g

12. 5 mg = _____ g

13. 3000 mg = _____ g

14. 1500 mg = _____ g

15. 15,000 mg = _____ g

16. 10 mg = _____ g

17. 100 mg = _____ g

18. 0.5 mg = _____ g

19. 7.5 mg = _____ g

20. 20.15 mg = _____ g

Ratio and proportion

RULE: **1** To solve metric problems, first analyze the problem.

EXAMPLE: 40 mg = _____ g

You already know you can move the decimal point 3 places to the left (divide) and come out with the correct answer. However, now it's time to start setting up a ratio and proportion problem.

1 What we *know* goes on the *left*.

2 What we *want to know* (the *x,* or unknown) goes on the *right*.

Know	Want to know

1 g:1000 mg::x g:40 mg   PROOF: $1000 \times 0.04 = 40$

$1000x = 40$ $1 \times 40 = 40$

$$\frac{\cancel{1000}x}{\cancel{1000}} = \frac{40}{1000} = 40 \div 1000$$

$$\begin{array}{r} .04 \\ 1000\overline{)40.00} \\ \underline{40\ 00} \end{array}$$

$x = 0.04$ g   Always *label* your answer.

3B # Worksheet   (Answers on p. 154)

Show all work, prove, and label all answers:

REMEMBER: 1 mg = 1000 μg

$\qquad\qquad$ 1 g = 1000 mg

$\qquad\qquad$ 1 kg (2.2 lb) = 1000 g

$\qquad\qquad$ 1 L = 1000 ml

Use ratio and proportion:

1. 25 mg = _____ g

2. 0.064 g = _____ mg

3. 4 mg = _____ g

4. 4.6 g = _____ mg

5. 375 ml = _____ L

6. 89 kg = _____ g

7. 45 mg = _____ g

8. 0.6 g = _____ mg

9. 50 kg = _____ lb

10. 2500 g = _____ lb

Two-step problems

MUST KNOW

$1000 \mu g = 1$ mg
1000 mg $= 1$ g
1000 g $= 1$ kg
1000 ml $= 1$ L

Two-step ratio and proportion

EXAMPLE: The doctor ordered 10 mg. On hand you have tablets of 0.002 g each. How many tablets will you give?

Step 1: Have g on hand. Need to change mg to g because that is what is on hand. What do you know about g and mg?

Know   Want to know

1000 mg:1 g::10 mg:x g

*Cancel x out:

PROOF: $1000 \times 0.01 = 10$

$1 \times 10 = 10$

$$\frac{\cancel{1000}x}{\cancel{1000}} = \frac{10}{1000} = 10 \div 1000 = 0.01$$

$x = 0.01$ g

The doctor ordered 10 mg. We now know that 10 mg $= 0.01$ g. Now set up the second step to solve the problem.

Step 2: **Know**   **Want to know**

   0.002 g:1 tab.::0.01 g:x tab.   PROOF: $0.002 \times 5 = 0.01$

   *Cancel x out: $1 \times 0.01 = 0.01$

$$\frac{0.002x}{0.002} = \frac{0.01}{0.002} = 0.01 \div 0.002 = 5$$

   $x = 5$ tab. of 0.002 g each

3C **Worksheet**   (Answers on p. 156)

Two-step metric problems. Show all work, set up ratio and proportion, prove, and label all work. Remember to estimate your answer when you reach the second step.

1. Doctor ordered 0.75 g of erythromycin. On hand you have 250 mg tablets. How many tablets will you give?

2. Doctor ordered Valium 10 mg. On hand you have Valium 0.005 g tablets. How many tablets will you give?

3. Ordered is 3 mg of codeine. On hand you have 0.002 g tablets of codeine. How many tablets will you give?

4. Doctor ordered 75 mg of Demerol IM. On hand you have a vial of 0.050 g per ml. How many ml will you give?

---

*There is no need to cancel out if you make sure to put the x on the *left* side and remember to divide the x into the sum on the *right* side of the equation.

5. Doctor ordered chlorpromazine 0.075 g. On hand you have chlorpromazine 25 mg/ml. How many ml will you give?

6. Ordered is 2 g of Staphcillin. The vial reads: "Add 8.6 ml of diluent to contents of vial. Each ml will contain 500 mg of Staphcillin." How many ml will you administer?

7. Doctor ordered 500 mg of Gantrisin. Available are Gantrisin 0.25 g tablets. How many tablets will you give?

8. You are to give 0.125 g of Keflin. On hand you have Keflin 50 mg/5 ml. How many ml will you give? The Keflin will be administered in an IV solution.

9. Doctor ordered Robinul 0.002 g. Available are 1-mg tablets. How many tablets will you give?

10. Ordered is 2 mg of verapamil hydrochloride IV. On hand you have 5 mg/2 ml. How many ml will you give?

■ Metric System Test   (Answers on p. 159)

Use ratio and proportion. Estimate your answer; label and prove answer.

1. 500 mg = _____ g

2. 25 mg = _____ g

3. 5 mg = _____ g

4. 0.2 g = _____ mg

5. 4 g = _____ mg

6. Doctor ordered 10 mg of Valium. On hand you have 0.02 g in each tablet. How many tablets will you give? (Is this a one-step or a two-step problem?) Prove.

7. Doctor ordered 60 mg. On hand you have 20 mg tablets. How many tablets will you give? (Is this a one-step or a two-step problem?)

8. Ordered is 0.75 g. On hand you have 250 mg tablets. How many tablets will you give? (Is this a one-step or two-step problem?)

9. Doctor ordered 500 mg of Achromycin. On hand are 250 mg tablets. You will give _____ tablets.

10. Digitoxin 0.125 mg tablets are on hand. Give 0.25 mg. How many tablets will you give?

Apothecary system

Objectives

- *Memorize symbols for dram, ounce, drop, and minim.*
- *Calculate one-step apothecary system problems.*

Explanation

The apothecary system is an imprecise old English system of measurement that is not being used very often today. The metric system has virtually replaced the apothecary system. The apothecary system is written in fractions and Roman numerals. This system does not convert exactly to other systems of measurement.

Household

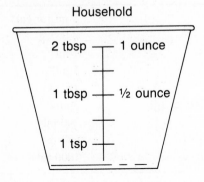

Apothecary

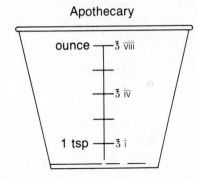

Metric

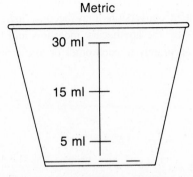

One ounce medicine cups (30 ml)

■ VOLUME (WET) ■

gtt = drop = minim (m, ɱ, or m)
60 minims (m) = 1 dram (dr or ℨ) = 1 tsp = 5 ml = 60 gtt
1 ounce (oz or ℥) = 30 ml = 8 tsp
16 oz (℥) = 1 pint (pt or O) = 500 ml
2 pt = 1 quart (qt) = 1000 ml
4 qt = 1 gallon (gal or C) = 4000 ml
32 oz (℥) = 1 qt = 1000 ml

MUST KNOW:
ℨ = dram (dr)
℥ = ounce (oz)
gtt = drop
m = minim

Equivalents

■ Table 1. Approximate equivalents of metric, apothecary, and household measures

Household	Apothecary	Metric
60 drops (gtt)	1 teaspoon (tsp)	5 ml (or cc)*
1 drop (gtt)	1 minim	0.065 g
	15 or 16 minims	1 ml
1 teaspoon (tsp)	1 fluidram (ℨ)	5 ml
1 tablespoon (tbs)	4 fluidrams	15 ml
2 tablespoons (tbs)	8 fluidrams = 1 ounce (℥)	30 ml
1 measuring cup	8 ounces	240 ml
1 pint	1 pint or 16 ounces	500 ml
1 quart	1 quart or 32 ounces	1000 ml

*The abbreviations *ml* and *cc* are used interchangeably; however, *ml* should be used for liquids, *cc* for solids and gases, and *g* for solids.

NOTE: Household measurement conversions may become increasingly important with the trend toward home health care. Also, the apothecary measures and household teaspoons, drams, and tablespoons do not convert accurately to each other or to metric measurements.

Roman numerals and Arabic numerals

Roman numerals are used with the apothecary system. Usually Arabic numerals are used for numbers over 9. Fractions are written with Arabic numerals except for $\overline{ss}$ (semis), which stands for one half. If the quantity is composed of a whole number and a fraction, the entire amount is written in Arabic numerals.

Arabic numerals	Capital roman numerals	Small roman numerals
1	I	i
2	II	ii
3	III	iii
4	IV	iv
5	V	v
6	VI	vi
7	VII	vii
8	VIII	viii
9	IX	ix
10	X	x
19	XIX	xix
20	XX	xx
30	XXX	xxx
40	XL	xl
49	XLIX	xlix
50	L	l
60	LX	lx
70	LXX	lxx
80	LXXX	lxxx
90	XC	xc
100	C	c
500	D	d
1000	M	m

In the apothecary system the measure or symbol precedes the number. The abbreviation *gr* means grain (originally a grain of wheat).

EXAMPLE: gr xv, gr XV
                ʒ i (in handwriting: ʒ ī)
                ℥ ii (in handwriting: ℥ īi)
                gr $\overline{ss}$ (one half)
                gtt ii (drops)

NOTE: Don't confuse ʒ (dram) and ℥ (ounce).

Ratio and proportion

EXAMPLE: You have a vial of caffeine containing gr 1½ per ml. Doctor ordered caffeine gr 3¾. How many ml will you give?

What was ordered and what you *have* on hand are in the same system; therefore, it is a one-step problem.

REMEMBER: *Have* or *know* goes on the *left*.

Have   **Want to know**

gr 1½:1 ml::gr 3¾:x ml

$$\frac{1\frac{1}{2}x}{1\frac{1}{2}} = \frac{3\frac{3}{4}}{1\frac{1}{2}} = \frac{15}{4} \div \frac{3}{2} = \frac{15}{4} \times \frac{2}{3} = \frac{30}{12} = 2\frac{1}{2}$$

$x = 2\frac{1}{2}$ ml = 2.5 ml

PROOF: $1 \times 3\frac{3}{4} = 3\frac{3}{4}$

$1\frac{1}{2} \times 2\frac{1}{2} = 3\frac{3}{4}$

4A Worksheet   (Answers on p. 159)

Using ratio and proportion, prove:

1. You are to give codeine gr i. You have codeine gr s̄s̄ per ml. How many ml will you give?

2. You are to give ASA gr XV. You have ASA gr V per tablet. How many tablets will you give?

3. Doctor ordered morphine sulfate gr ⅙. You have on hand a vial containing morphine sulfate gr ⅛ per ml. How many ml will you give? (For amounts over 1 ml, calculate to tenths; for amounts under 1 ml, calculate to hundredths.)

4. Doctor ordered an aminophylline suppository gr XV. On hand you have aminophylline suppository gr vīīs̄s̄. How many suppositories will you give?

5. On hand you have a can of Metamucil containing ℥ viii. You are to give Metamucil ʒ ii. How many teaspoons will you mix with juice or water? How many ml is this?

6. You are to give ʒ ss of Maalox. On hand you have a bottle containing Maalox ℥ viii. How many ml will you give?

7. You are to give codeine sulfate gr ⅙ SC. On hand you have codeine sulfate gr ¼ per ml. How many ml will you give? Your immediate reaction will be to give _____ (more or less) than 1 ml. (Calculate to hundredths. Do not round.)

8. You are to give Nembutal gr iss. On hand you have Nembutal gr ss. How many capsules will you give?

9. Doctor ordered amobarbital sodium gr iii IV. You have gr ii per 1.25 ml sterile water. Will you give more or less than 1.25 ml? How many ml will you give? (*Hint:* Be sure all your numbers are in decimals OR fractions. Don't mix the two.)

10. Doctor ordered Seconal gr iii. On hand you have Seconal capsules gr iss. How many capsules will you give?

Worksheet   (Answers on p. 162)

1. Doctor ordered morphine sulfate gr ⅛. On hand you have a vial containing morphine sulfate gr ¹⁄₁₀ per ml. How many minims will you give?

2. Doctor ordered Robitussin ℥ ¼. How many drams (℈) will you give?

3. Doctor ordered atropine gr ¹⁄₂₀₀. On hand you have an ampule of atropine labeled gr ¹⁄₁₅₀ per 0.5 ml. How many ml will you give? How many minims will you give?

4. On hand you have Gantrisin tablets gr V. Doctor ordered Gantrisin tablets gr 15. How many tablets will you give?

5. Doctor ordered ℥ s̄s̄ of cough syrup. How many drams is this? How many ml will you give?

■ Apothecary System Test   (Answers on p. 163)

1. Doctor has ordered Pantopon gr ⅙ IM q.4h. p.r.n. The vial on hand is labeled Pantopon gr ⅓ in 1 ml. How much will you give?

2. You are to give atropine gr ¹⁄₂₀₀ as a preoperative medication. The vial on hand is labeled gr ¹⁄₁₅₀ in 1 ml solution. How many ml will you give?

3. You are to give morphine sulfate gr ⅙ with the above atropine. The morphine available is labeled gr ¼ in 1 ml. How many ml will you give?

4. Doctor has ordered elixir of terpin hydrate (ETH) with codeine ʒ iii. This is equal to how many ml?

5. You are to give codeine gr ⅛. The drug available is labeled codeine gr ¼ per ml. How many ml will you give?

6. You are to give atropine gr ½00. On hand is a Tubex cartridge with gr ⅟₁₅₀ in 0.5 ml. How many ml will you give? How many minims is this?

7. You have a vial of caffeine containing gr 1½ per ml. You are to give gr ¾. How many ml will you give?

8. You are to give Gantrisin gr XV. On hand are Gantrisin tablets gr V. How many tablets will you give?

9. You have Tuinal gr s̄s̄ capsules on hand. Doctor has ordered Tuinal gr i̇. How many capsules will you give?

10. Doctor ordered Seconal gr ı̇ı̇ı̇. On hand you have Seconal gr ı̄s̄s̄ capsules. How many capsules will you give?

Apothecary and metric conversions

Objectives

- *Calculate milligram/grain/gram equivalencies.*

- *Calculate milliliter/quart/liter/pint and dram/minim/ounce equivalencies.*

- *Round minims and drops to nearest correct number.*

- *Convert grains/grams/milligrams by using one-step ratio and proportion method.*

- *Calculate metric-apothecary conversion problems.*

Equivalency tables

■ VOLUME ■

1000 milliliters (ml) = 1 liter (L) = 1 quart (qt)

1 ml = 1 cubic centimeter (cc)

500 ml = 1 pint (pt)

30 ml = 1 ounce (℥) or 8 drams (ʒ)

5 ml = 1 dram = 1 tsp = 4 or 5 ml

1 ml = 15 or 16 minims (℩)

1 m̄ = 1 drop (gtt)

■ WEIGHT ■

1000 mg = 1 gram (g) = gr XV (15)

500 mg = 0.5 g = gr VIISS

60–67* mg = gr i̇

0.6 mg = gr 1/100

0.4 mg = gr 1/150

0.3 mg = gr 1/200

*The value 60 mg is more commonly used (see diagram next page). The value gr 1/60 = 1 mg is more commonly used than gr 1/67.

Apothecary system does not convert exactly to metric.

A GOOD WAY TO REMEMBER:

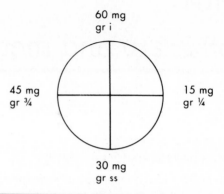

"The Metric Clock"

(Clock diagram labels)
60 mg
gr i

45 mg
gr ¾

15 mg
gr ¼

30 mg
gr ss

RULE 1: When working with decimals, always remember to add a zero if there is no number before the decimal. This clarifies the decimal position and prevents medication errors.

EXAMPLE: 0.1 g is different from 1.0 g.

RULE 2: Apothecary is made definitive by adding a dot for clarification of the number one.

EXAMPLE: gr i (1) or gr viiss (7½)

RULE 3: When working with the metric system, note that the symbol *follows* the Arabic number.

EXAMPLE: 0.5 g

RULE 4: When working with the apothecary system, note that Roman numerals are frequently used. The symbol *precedes* the number.

EXAMPLE: gr xv

When proving answers from apothecary to metric, you will notice a slight difference (one tenth) because the apothecary system is not so accurate as the metric system. Proving answers *must* be done with the original answer and then rounded off if necessary.

EXAMPLE: **Know**   **Want to know**
1.0 g:gr 15::x g:gr 5   PROOF: $1.0 \times 5 = 5$
$15x = 5$ $15 \times 0.33 = 4.95 = 5$
$x = 0.333$ g

Rounding Off

EXAMPLE: **Minims**   11.6   Give 12 ♏.
              Drops   6.7 gtt   Give 7 gtt.

Syringes are calibrated in minims and tenths as well as ml. Therefore if the answer is 1.7 ml, do NOT round off to 2 ml. Tenths and hundredths can be measured accurately on syringes.

EXAMPLE: 1.68 ml   Give 1.7 ml in a 2 or 3 ml syringe.

The 8 in 1.68 is greater than 5, so the next highest number can be added to the 6, making the correct dosage 1.7 ml.

EXAMPLE: 0.73 ml   Give 0.73 ml.

Use a TB syringe for amounts less than 1 ml when a very precise dosage is indicated.

5A Worksheet   (Answers on p. 164)

MEMORIZE: 1 g = gr 15
          60 mg = gr i

One-step problems

Use ratio and proportion, prove answers, and label answers:

1. gr 10 = _____ g

2. 0.5 g = gr _____

3. gr xxx = _____ g

4. 0.1 g = gr _____

5. gr viiss = _____ g

6. 3.0 g = gr _____

7. gr ¾ = _____ mg

8. 60 mg = gr _____

9. gr ¼ = _____ mg

10. gr $\frac{1}{150}$ = _____ mg

Worksheet   (Answers on p. 165)

Figure these in your head. Complete the following equivalents:

1. 1 mg = _____ g

2. 5 g = _____ mg

3. 1 g = gr _____

4. gr 7½ = _____ g

5. 15 mg = gr _____

6. 1 L = _____ ml

7. 30 ml = _____ ʒ

8. 1 ml = _____ gtt

9. 2 ʒ = _____ ml

10. 1 cc = _____ ml

11. 1 kg = _____ g

12. gr $^1/_{200}$ = _____ mg

13. gr iii = _____ mg

14. ʒ i = _____ ml

15. 1 tsp = _____ ml

16. 1 gtt = _____ ℔

17. Which is smaller: mg or gr? _____

18. Which is larger: g or gr? _____

19. Which is larger: 30 ml or ½ oz? _____

20. Which is larger: 15 ml or ʒ? _____

5C **Worksheet**   (Answers on p. 165)

MUST KNOW:

1 g = gr 15
gr i = 60 mg
ʒ i = 30 ml
1 ml = 15 to 16 ℔
ʒ i = 5 ml

1. You are to give Milk of Magnesia (MOM) ʒ iss. How many ml will you give?

2. Doctor ordered atropine sulfate gr ⅟₃₀₀ to be given on call to the O.R. On hand you have 0.50 mg per 0.5 ml. How many ml will you give?

3. You need to give Robitussin ℨ ii p.o. How many ml will you give?

4. Doctor ordered Demerol gr ¾. On hand you have a vial of Demerol labeled 75 mg/cc. How many ml will you give?

5. You are to give ASA (acetylsalicylic acid) 0.6 g. The tablets on hand are labeled ASA gr v. How many tablets will you give?

6. Doctor ordered 720 mg ASA for a temperature above 101° F. Your patient developed a fever of 101° F. How many tablets of ASA gr 5 per tablet will you give?

7. You are to give caffeine sodium benzoate gr viiss. You have an ampule labeled caffeine sodium benzoate 0.5 g in 2.0 cc. How many ml will you give?

8. You have a 2-ml ampule of caffeine Na benzoate containing gr viiss. If the physician orders gr V, how many ml will you give?

9. Doctor ordered Nembutal 100 mg. On hand you have Nembutal gr iss. How many capsules will you give?

10. You have an ampule of Amytal Sodium gr ii/1.25 ml on hand. Doctor ordered 30 mg IV. How many ml will you give?

5D Worksheet (Answers on p. 168)

1. The physician ordered gr ¹⁄₂₀₀ scopolamine SC injection. On hand is a vial of scopolamine that reads 1 ml = gr ¹⁄₁₅₀. How many ml would you give?

2. In the narcotic box the morphine is labeled M.S. gr ¼ per 1 cc. The physician ordered M.S. gr ⅙. How many ml would you give (to nearest tenth)?
   Before you begin this problem, can you tell if you will give more or less than 1 ml?

3. The physician ordered codeine gr ½ oral. On hand are 15-mg tablets. How many tablets would you give?

4. Penicillin 300,000 U IM is ordered every 4 hours. On hand is a 10-ml vial of penicillin labeled 400,000 U per 1 ml. How many minims would you give for 1 dose?

5. Gantrisin 0.50 g (oral) is ordered. On hand is Gantrisin 250 mg per tablet. How many tablets would you give?

6. Demerol 75 mg IM is ordered stat. On hand is Demerol 100 mg per 2 ml. How many ml would you give (nearest tenth)?

7. Atropine gr ¹⁄₃₀₀ by injection is ordered for a patient going to surgery. The nurse has a bottle from stock labeled scopolamine gr ¹⁄₁₅₀. How many minims of scopolamine would you give?

8. Chloral hydrate gr viiss is ordered for sleep. On hand is a bottle marked chloral hydrate. One tablet is 0.25 g. How many tablets would you give?

9. MOM with cascara ℥ ss is ordered. How many ml will you give?

10. Morphine gr ¹⁄₂₀₀ IM is ordered. On hand you have an ampule labeled morphine 0.4 mg per ml. How many ml will you give?

Prove and label answers:

1. Atropine gr $\frac{1}{150}$ per ml is found in stock. The physician ordered gr $\frac{1}{200}$ to be given by injection. How many minims would you give?

2. Maalox is ordered ℥ s̄s̄ q.2h. How many ml would you give? How many ml will you give in 24 hours?

3. Ordered was tincture of belladonna minims IX in ½ glass water. How many drops would you use?

4. How many ml of water would you use for the preceding if the glass holds 6 oz?

5. Elixir of phenobarbital 8 ml was ordered. How many teaspoons is this? How many ℥ is this?

6. The physician ordered Kantrex 0.2 g q.4h. by injection. The vial of Kantrex is labeled "Add 5 ml sterile water for 1 g per 2 ml." How many ml would you give?

7. Ordered was 0.05 g Talwin p.o. On hand were 100 mg tablets of Talwin. How many tablets will you give?

8. Ordered was 15 mg of Vasotec. On hand are 0.03 g tablets of Vasotec. How many tablets will you give?

9. Captopril 0.05 g was ordered. You have Captopril 25 mg tablets. How many tablets will you give?

10. Cefaclor 0.1 g was ordered. On hand you have 125 mg/5 ml. How many ml will you give?

■ Apothecary and Metric Conversions Test   (Answers on p. 172)

Use ratio and proportion, prove, and label:

1. gr 10 = _____ g

5. gr 5 = _____ g

2. 0.5 g = gr _____

6. gr viiss = _____ g

3. gr xxx = _____ g

7. 3 g = gr _____

4. 90 mg = gr _____

8. Ordered: tincture of belladonna minims ix in ½ glass water. How many drops will you give?

9. Ordered: morphine sulfate gr ⅙. On hand: morphine sulfate gr ¼ ml. Give _____ ml.

10. Ordered: atropine gr ⅟₃₀₀. On hand: atropine gr ⅟₁₅₀ per 0.5 ml. Give _____ ml.

CHAPTER 6

Medications from powder and crystals

Objectives

- *Reconstitute medications from powders and crystals.*
- *Determine the best dilution strength to mix for the ordered amount of medication.*

Explanation

Diluting powder or crystals in vials

Directions for dissolving drugs in vials can be found in the accompanying literature. Information given will be the volume of the powder after it is dissolved in NS or distilled water. For instance, the directions may read: "Add 1.4 ml NS to make 2 ml of reconstituted solution." These directions tell the user that the powder takes up to 0.6 ml of space.

$$1.4 \text{ ml} + 0.6 \text{ ml} = 2 \text{ ml}$$

> **RULE:** Read the label to find out how many units, grams, milligrams, or micrograms are in each ml of the reconstituted drug.

EXAMPLE: DIRECTIONS: Add 1.4 ml distilled water (sterile) to make 600,000 U of penicillin per 2 ml.

Ordered: 300,000 U penicillin IM q.6h.

Have	Want
2 ml:600,000 U::x ml:300,000 U	PROOF: $2 \times 3 = 6$
$6x = 6$	$6 \times 1 = 6$
$x = 1$ ml	

Give 1 ml of reconstituted solution for each 300,000 U.

Many solutions are unstable after being reconstituted. Read directions carefully for storing in the refrigerator or in a dark place. There is usually a time limit or expiration date on the vial. It is important to date, label, and initial all reconstituted medications.

Worksheet (Answers on p. 172)

1. Ordered: Kefzol (cefazolin sodium) 300 mg IM.
   - How many ml of diluent will be used?
   - How many mg/ml will it make?
   - What is the shelf life of the medication after reconstitution?
   - How many ml will you give?

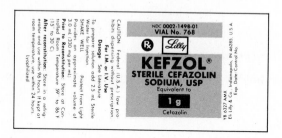

2. Ordered: Prostaphlin 450 mg IM.
   - How many ml of sterile water for injection will be used?
   - How many mg/ml will it make?
   - What is the shelf life of the medication after reconstitution?
   - How many ml will you give?

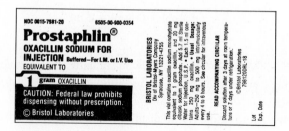

3. Ordered: 500 mg Polycillin-N IM q.6h.
   - How many ml of diluent are needed to reconstitute?
   - How many mg/ml will it make?
   - What is the shelf life of the medication?
   - How many ml will you give?

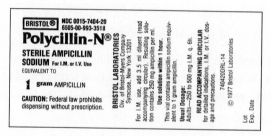

4. Ordered: 300 mg Prostaphlin IM q.4h.
   - How many ml of diluent should be used to reconstitute?
   - How many mg/ml will it make?
   - What is the shelf life of the medication?
   - How many ml will you give?

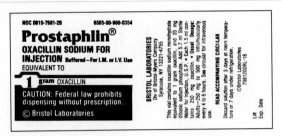

5. Ordered: 1000 mg Staphcillin IM q.6h.
   - How many ml of diluent should be used to reconstitute?
   - How many g/ml will it make?
   - What is the shelf life of the medication?
   - How many ml of medication will you give?

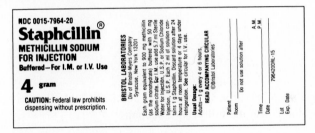

6. Ordered: Penicillin G Potassium 750,000 U IM.
   - Which strength will you use?
   - How many ml of diluent will be used?
   - What is the shelf life of the medication after reconstitution?
   - How many ml of medication will you give?

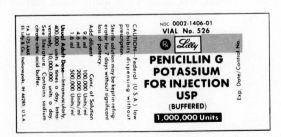

7. Ordered: 750 mg Ticar IM.
   - How many ml of diluent will be added?
   - How many g/ml will it make?
   - What is the shelf life of the medication?
   - How many ml will you give?

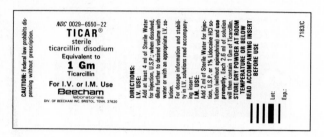

6B Worksheet (Answers on p. 173)

1. Ordered: Prostaphlin (sodium oxacillin) 500 mg IM. You have a multidose vial that reads: "Prostaphlin; add 5.7 ml sterile water for injection." Each 1.5 ml of solution contains 0.25 g. How many ml will you give?

2. Ordered: potassium penicillin G (Pfizerpen) 300,000 U IM. You have a multidose vial containing 1 million U and the following directions:

Ml of diluent added	Units per ml
19.6	50,000
9.6	100,000
3.6	250,000
1.6	500,000

Which dilution will you make and label? How many ml or part of ml will you give?

3. Ordered: 200 mg Keflin IM q.4h. Available is Keflin (cephalothin sodium) 1 g in a 10 ml vial. Each g of Keflin should be diluted with 4 ml of sterile water for injection. The reconstituted material will provide two 500-mg doses of 2.2 ml each. How many ml will you give?

4. Ordered: 125 mg Kefzol (cefazolin sodium) IM. Available is cefazolin sodium 500 mg with the following directions for reconstitution: ''Add 2 ml sterile water for injection or 0.9% sodium chloride for injection. Provides approximate volume of 2.2 ml (225 mg/ml) after reconstitution. Store in refrigerator. Protect from light, and use within 96 hours. If kept at room temperature, use within 24 hours.'' How many ml will you give?

5. Ordered: Totacillin-N (sodium ampicillin) 500 mg IM stat. Available is a powdered form labeled ''0.50 g for IV or IM use. For IM use, add at least 1.7 ml sterile water for injection, USP. Use solution within 1 hour after reconstituting.'' Each ml will contain 0.25 g. How many ml will you give?

6. Ordered: Achromycin V 500 mg IV volutrol stat. Available is Achromycin (tetracycline hydrochloride) 0.50 g for IV administration only. Directions: ''Add 10 ml of sterile water for injection. After solution has been prepared, it should be further diluted to at least 100 ml (up to 1000 ml) prior to administration.'' How many ml will you dilute in the IV volutrol bag, which holds 100 ml?

7. Ordered: Kantrex (kanamycin sulfate) 300 mg IM. Direct[i] sterile water for injection to make 1 g per 3 ml.'' After re[give?

8. Ordered: 1.2 million units of penicillin. You have a 10 ml vial containing 0.5 million U/ml. How many ml will you give? How many ml will be left in the vial? How many units of penicillin will be left in the vial?

9. A vial of penicillin contains 5 million U. Doctor ordered 500,000 U. You wish to make each ml equal 500,000 U. How many ml of diluent will you use?

10. A vial is labeled 500,000 U/ml. Doctor ordered 800,000 U IM q.4h. How many ml will you give?

■ Medications From Powder and Crystals Test   (Answers on p. 175)

1. Doctor ordered penicillin G 300,000 U IM q.4h. Pharmacy sent a vial with 3 million U penicillin G in dry crystal form. Directions were to dilute with 4.2 ml NS to make 5 ml. After dilution, the vial contains 3 million units per 5 ml U. How many ml will you give?

2. Ordered: Keflin 0.5 g IM q.6h. Pharmacy sent a vial of sodium cephalothin (Keflin) 1 g in powder form. Directions read: "Add 4 ml sterile water to make two 0.5 g doses of 2.2 ml each." How many ml will you give?

3. Dilute a vial containing 500,000 U of Polycillin (ampicillin) so that each ml contains 50,000 U. How much distilled water will you need to add to the vial to get 50,000 U/ml?

4. A vial contains 1 million units of carbenicillin. Prepare the dry powder to contain a solution of 250,000 U/ml. How much distilled water will you need to add to the vial?

5. Doctor ordered 400,000 U Keflin. You have a vial with 600,000 U/ml. How many ml will you give?

CHAPTER 7

Insulin

Objective

■ *Convert insulin units to hundredths or tenths of a milliliter.*

> **RULE:** Use insulin syringes. If none are available, use a tuberculin syringe. Use ratio and proportion to convert your order from units to hundredths.

Explanation

The value and purity of drugs from animal sources vary. Therefore some hormones, such as insulin and heparin, are supplied in *units* (U), a standardized measurement based on strength rather than weight. You already know that insulin is an aqueous solution of the active principal hormone of the pancreas. It affects the metabolism of glucose. Insulin comes from animal sources of beef, pork pancreas, and recombinant DNA techniques (Humulin).

Insulin is supplied in units and is given with special insulin syringes. Most commonly, insulin is supplied in 10-ml vials labeled U 100, which means 100 U/ml. Insulin is also supplied in 10-ml vials labeled "U 500," which means 500 U/ml.* This strength is used for diabetic patients whose blood sugar fluctuates to very high levels. The concentrated solution of 500 U/ml allows a concentrated dose in less fluid, avoiding the pain of large fluid injections.

Because many patients require insulin injections on a regular basis, it is important to use multiple injection sites and to plan the rotation schedule (Fig. 1).

Syringes

Insulin is usually given in a 1-ml or 0.5-ml insulin syringe calibrated to U 100 insulin. Insulin can also be given in a tuberculin syringe as it is calibrated on 100 (Fig. 2). The 0.5-ml insulin syringe is used for smaller doses, as the calibrations are larger and easier to read.

---

*For brittle diabetes.

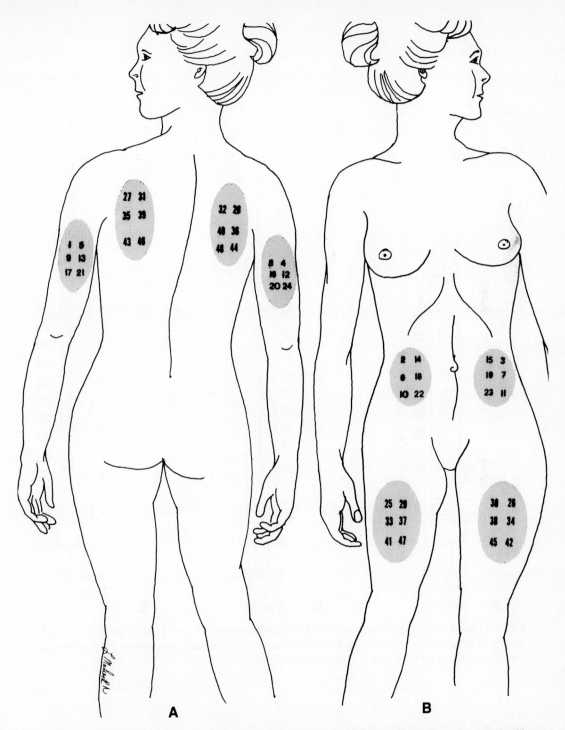

Fig. 1. Subcutaneous injection sites and rotation plan. **A,** Posterior view. **B,** Anterior view. (From Clayton, B.D., et al.: Squire's basic pharmacology for nurses, ed. 8, St. Louis, 1985, The C.V. Mosby Co.)

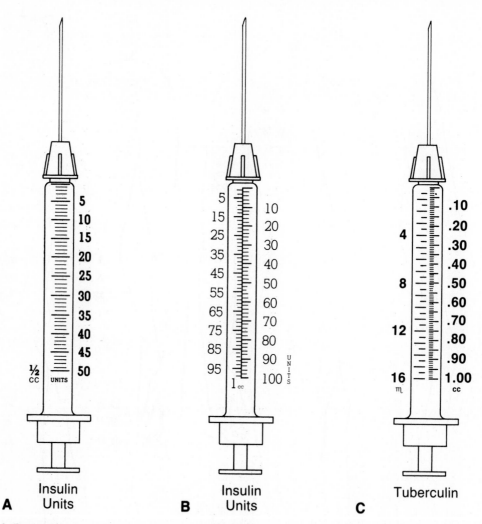

Fig. 2. Types of syringes. **A,** Insulin units. Each calibration represents 1 unit. Used for smaller doses of U 100 insulin. **B,** Insulin units. Each calibration represents 2 units. **C,** Tuberculin (16 minim = 1 ml). Minims on one side, graduated on the other side in 0.01 (hundredths) ml.

A typical order for insulin must include:

    a. The *name* of the insulin: regular, lente, NPH, etc.

    b. The *number* of units the patient will receive: regular insulin 10 U.

    c. The *time* to be given: regular insulin 10 U, in AM, ½ hr a.c.

    d. The *strength* to be given: regular insulin U 100, 10 U, in AM, ½ hr a.c.

EXAMPLE: **1** Give 30 units of U 100 insulin using a U 100 syringe. Fill syringe to the 30 U calibration. Always have another registered nurse check the order, label, and dosage before administering. For U 500, have *two* nurses check.

EXAMPLE: **2** Doctor ordered regular insulin U 100, 30 U in AM ½ hour before meals. There are no U 100 syringes. Use ratio and proportion: You know that U 100 insulin has 100 U in 1 ml.*

Have   **Want**

100 U : 1 ml :: 30 U : x ml   PROOF: $100 \times 0.3 = 30$

$$\frac{100x}{100} = \frac{1 \times 30}{100} = \frac{30}{100} = \frac{3}{10}$$ $1 \times 30 = 30$

$x = 0.3$ ml of U 100 insulin in a 3-ml syringe and 0.3-ml in a tuberculin syringe

Types of insulin

Short-acting (peaks first shift)

    1. Regular

    2. Semilente

    3. Humulin R

Intermediate-acting (peaks second shift)

    1. NPH (neutral protamine)

    2. Lente

    3. Globin

    4. Humulin N

Long-acting (peaks third shift)

    1. PZI (protamine zinc insulin)

    2. Ultralente

    3. Humulin L

---

*Tuberculin syringes are calibrated in hundredths and tenths.

Carry out to two decimal places (hundredths):

1. Convert 15 units of U 100 to ml.

2. Convert 75 units of U 100 to ml.

3. Convert 150 units of U 500 to ml.

4. Convert 45 units of U 100 to ml.

5. Ordered: regular insulin U 100 daily in AM. What is the matter with this order?

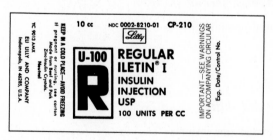

6. Ordered: Lente insulin porcine U 100 q.AM. (*Porcine* means insulin is from pork pancreas, and bottle is labeled that way.) What would you question about this order?

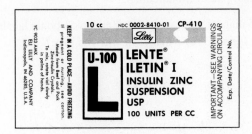

7. Ordered: NPH 100 units of insulin daily in AM. How many ml would your patient need if you used U 100 insulin?

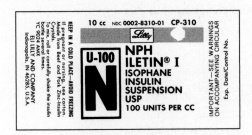

8. Ordered: Lente insulin 34 U SC q.AM. Available is a 0.5-ml insulin syringe. How many units will you measure?

9. Ordered: Regular insulin 20 U and Lente humulin insulin 36 U SC q.AM. Available is a U 100 insulin syringe. What is the total amount to be given?

10. Ordered: Ultralente 18 U and Humulin regular 16 U. Available is a TB syringe. How many ml of Ultralente will you measure? How many ml of Humulin R will you measure? How many total ml will you give?

Carry out to two decimal places (hundredths):

1. You are to give 35 units of regular insulin. You have a bottle labeled regular insulin U 100 and a 1-ml tuberculin syringe. How many ml will you give?

2. Ordered: 20 units of regular insulin a.c. t.i.d.
   On hand: regular insulin U 100

   How many ml would you give? _____

3. Ordered: Lente 45 units q.d.
   On hand: Lente U 100

   How many ml will you give? _____

4. Ordered: regular insulin 65 units.
   Available: regular insulin U 100 containing 100 U/ml

   How many ml will you give? _____

5. Ordered: 20 units of regular insulin stat.
   Available: U 100 regular insulin

   You will give _____ ml.

6. Ordered: NPH insulin 40 units SC every AM ½ hr a.c.
   Available: NPH insulin U 100

   How many ml will you give? _____

7. Ordered: regular insulin 160 units.
   Available: regular insulin U 500

   You will give _____ ml.

8. Ordered: PZI insulin 15 U SC with 20 U regular insulin q.AM. Use a tuberculin syringe. How many total ml will you give? How many m̅ is this?

9. Ordered: Semilente insulin 25 U SC q.AM. Using a TB syringe, how many ml will you give?

10. Ordered: Ultralente insulin 30 units q.AM. Using an insulin syringe, measure 30 units.

■ Insulin Test   (Answers on p. 178)

Carry out to 2 decimal places (hundredths):

1. Ordered: regular insulin 65 units deep SC stat.
   Available: regular insulin U 100 and no insulin syringe. How many ml will you give?

2. Ordered: regular insulin 4 units a.c., q.AM.
   Available: regular insulin U 100 and no insulin syringe. How many ml will you give?

3. Ordered: regular insulin 16 units with NPH insulin 30 units a.c. q.AM.
   Available: regular insulin U 100 and NPH insulin U 100 and no insulin syringes.

   a. How many ml of regular insulin will you give?

   b. How many ml of NPH will you give?

4. Ordered: Lente insulin 18 U q.d.
   Available: Lente insulin U 100 and no insulin syringes. How many ml will you give?

5. Ordered: Humulin Lente insulin 16 U. Available is a tuberculin syringe. How many ml will you give?

CHAPTER 8

Heparin

Objective

■ *Convert heparin units to hundredths or tenths of a milliliter.*

Explanation

Sodium heparin injection, USP, is a drug used to interrupt the clotting process. It may be given in therapeutic dosages or in small diluted dosages to maintain the patency of IV or IA lines. Because it is inactive orally, sodium heparin is usually administered intravenously or subcutaneously. If administered intramuscularly, the drug produces a high level of pain and may cause hematomas. Sodium heparin is obtained commercially from domestic animals slaughtered for food. The orders for heparin are highly individualized and based on laboratory studies. Heparin comes in various strengths, that is, 5000 U/ml, 10,000 U/ml, 20,000 U/ml, and 50,000 U/ml.

The vial must be checked carefully before administration. Heparin is fast acting and may be counteracted with protamine sulfate. Check laboratory values for clotting times *before* administering heparin. Heparin orders, dosage, vial, and amount in syringe should be checked with another registered nurse.

Heparin is supplied in units, as is insulin, because the purity varies among sources. Heparin is often supplied in preprepared syringes. If you need to give less than the amount in the syringe, calculate the fractional amount you need to give and then transfer the heparin to a tuberculin syringe.*

RULE: The dosage of SC heparin should not exceed 1 ml.

EXAMPLE: ORDERED: Heparin 3500 U SC. On hand is a prepared vial containing 5000 U/ml. How many ml will you give?

Have   **Want**

5000 U:1 ml::3500 U:x ml

$5000x = 3500$

$x = 0.7$ ml

---

*The new syringe with sterile needle is advisable because the heparin inside the original needle may track through the subcutaneous tissue on insertion and cause bruising. Add 0.2 ml of air to syringe to ensure that all medication is administered, which will prevent tracking.

Worksheet   (Answers on p. 179)

Label and prove (carry out to nearest hundredths):

1. Give heparin 7000 U. On hand you have heparin 10,000 U/ml. How many ml will you give?

2. Ordered: 15,000 U heparin. How many ml will you give if you have heparin 20,000 U/ml?

3. Ordered: heparin 2500 U. On hand you have heparin 20,000 U/ml. How many ml will you give?

4. Ordered: heparin 17,000 U. On hand you have heparin 10,000 U/ml and 20,000 U/ml. Which strength will you choose? How many ml will you give?

5. Ordered: heparin 7500 U. How many ml will you give if the vial on hand reads heparin 10,000 U/ml?

■ Heparin Test   (Answers on p. 179)

1. Ordered: heparin 4000 U SC. The vial on hand is 5000 U/ml. How many ml will you give using a TB syringe?

2. Ordered: heparin 2500 U q.4h. SC. The vial on hand is labeled 10,000 U/ml. How many ml will you give using an insulin syringe?

3. Ordered: 2000 U heparin q.4h. SC. The vials on hand are 5000 U/ml and 10,000 U/ml. Which vial will you choose? Using a tuberculin syringe, how many ml will you give?

4. Ordered: 7000 U heparin q.6h. SC. The vials on hand are 5000 U/ml, 10,000 U/ml, and 20,000 U/ml. Which one will you choose? How many ml will you give?

5. Ordered: 3000 U heparin q.4h. SC. On hand is a vial of heparin 5000 U/ml. Using a tuberculin syringe, how many ml will you give?

CHAPTER 9

Children's dosages

Objectives

- *Estimate kilograms for given number of pounds.*
- *Calculate kilograms for given number of pounds.*
- *Calculate 24-hour dosages.*
- *Calculate safe dosage ranges in milligrams for given mg/kg formula and stated weight in pounds and ounces.*
- *Calculate pediatric dosage using BSA method.*
- *Calculate pediatric dosage using Clark's rule.*
- *Determine if pediatric drug order is within safe dosage range.*

Explanation

Almost all medications are calculated for the average adult dosage. Babies and children receive less medication. It is very important for the nurse to double check all physicians' medication orders for children and infants to be certain that the dosage ordered is safe. Emergency situations may require quick calculations to determine the exact amount of medication to give or to determine the amount of overdose taken by the child. Remember that the nurse is legally responsible for safe dosage administration even though the physician writes the order. Prompt clarification with the physician is important if the dosage is too low to be therapeutic or too high to be safe.

There are several formulas for estimating the therapeutic dose for children according to age, weight, and body surface area (BSA). The formulas for weight and body surface area are more accurate, and these are the methods that you will find in your references, the literature that accompanies the medication, and the *Physician's Desk Reference* (PDR).

Mg/kg method

The mg/kg method is the most frequently used means of calculating a therapeutic dose for pediatric medication administration. The literature accompanying most medications states the safe amount of drug in milligrams per kilogram of body weight for a 24-hour period. The amount of mg/kg is less for children than adults. You may also see μg/kg cited for therapeutic dose when very small amounts of medication will be given.

> **RULE:** Estimate, then calculate body weight in kg. Calculate the total mg permitted for that body weight. Compare the results with the physician's 24-hour order.* If the dose is safe, calculate and administer the dose ordered. If it is unsafe, hold and clarify.*

Steps to solving problems

1. Estimate the child's weight in kg by dividing the pounds in half (12 lb = approximately 6 kg). Always estimate your answers.

2. Calculate the child's exact weight in kg to two decimal places.† Note whether this calculation will be a one-step or two-step problem.

   a. If the child's weight is in ounces (for example, 8 lb, 6 oz), first convert the ounces to hundredths of a pound. Add this to the pounds, which will give total weight. Then convert the pounds (total) to kilograms. (This would be a two-step calculation.)

   b. If the child's weight is already in pounds only (for example, 8 lb), convert the pounds to kg. (This would be a one-step calculation.) Is your answer close to the estimate? (This is a safety check.)

3. Consult the literature for the safe pediatric range for this medication in mg/kg or μg/kg. Set up a ratio and proportion with the recommended mg/kg as the known and the x mg/child's weight in kg as the amount you want to know.

4. Compare the amount the physician has ordered for 24 hours with the safe amount determined by your calculations.* If the amount is safe, calculate the ordered dose of medication to be given. If it is unsafe, withhold the medication and clarify promptly with the physician.

---

*Be sure the two comparisons are for the same time periods.
†Calculate to hundredths.

EXAMPLE: Doctor ordered Lincocin 50 mg q.6h. IM. Baby weighs 12 lb, 6 oz today. On hand you have Lincocin 300 mg/ml. The literature states that the safe range is 20 mg/kg q.24h.*

- What is estimated weight in kg?
  12 ÷ 2 = 6 lb estimated weight

- What is exact weight in kg? A weight of 12 lb, 6 oz involves a two-step conversion.

Know	Want to know

a. 16 oz:1 lb::6 oz:x lb   PROOF: $16 \times 0.37 = 5.92$

$$\frac{\cancel{16}x}{\cancel{16}} = \frac{6}{16}$$
$$6 \times 1 = 6$$

Baby weighs 12.37 lb.

Know	Want to know

b. 2.2 lb:1 kg::12.37 lb:x kg

$$\frac{\cancel{2.2}x}{\cancel{2.2}} = \frac{12.37}{2.2}$$

$x = 5.62$ kg†

- What is the maximum recommended dose for this child's weight?

Know	Want to know

20 mg:1 kg::x mg:5.62 kg

$x = 20 \times 5.62$
$x = 112.4$ mg (safe 24-hour dosage)

- Is the order safe to give?
  No.

Doctor's order is 50 mg × 4, or 200 mg for 24 hours. Safe limit for this baby is 112 mg. The order exceeds the recommended dosage. Hold and clarify stat. Document. Unsafe order.

---

*Use *written* literature for medication references.
†Calculate kg to hundredths. Do not round.

BSA method (mg/m²)

The Body Surface Area (BSA) method is the most reliable way to calculate therapeutic dosages. It requires the use of a chart (nomogram) that converts weight to square meters (m²) of BSA. The average adult is assumed to weigh 140 lb and have 1.7 m² BSA. The BSA method is usually used to calculate safe doses for antineoplastic drugs,* new drugs, or drugs that normally aren't given to children. It is also used to determine therapeutic doses for underweight or overweight persons.

RULE: To determine the BSA (m²) of a child of normal height for weight, find the m² for that weight on the appropriate nomogram.

EXAMPLE: A child weighs 10 lb. Using the nomogram column for children of normal height for weight, a 10 lb child has a BSA of 0.27 m² (Fig. 3A).

EXAMPLE: A girl weighs 25 lb and is 32 inches (normal height for her weight). According to the nomogram (Fig. 3A) for children of normal height for weight, the BSA for 25 lb is 0.52.

RULE: To determine the BSA (m²) of a child who is underweight or overweight, find the m² for that weight by plotting the height in the height column and the weight in the weight column, using a straight line to join the two numbers. Where the line intersects on the surface area (SA) column is the m² for that child.

EXAMPLE: A 9 lb, 14 oz baby with a height of 60 cm would be underweight for height. Using a ruler to connect his height and weight, you would find a BSA of 0.28 m² (Fig. 3B).

---

*With antineoplastic therapy, doses are individualized on the basis of the severity of the illness, the kidney and renal function of the child, the response to therapy, individual versus multiple-dose therapy, and the sequence of the dose (first dose or later doses). Some doses for young children approach adult doses. Some tumors are now treated aggressively with "megadoses"—very large doses. When in doubt, clarify with the physician and document.

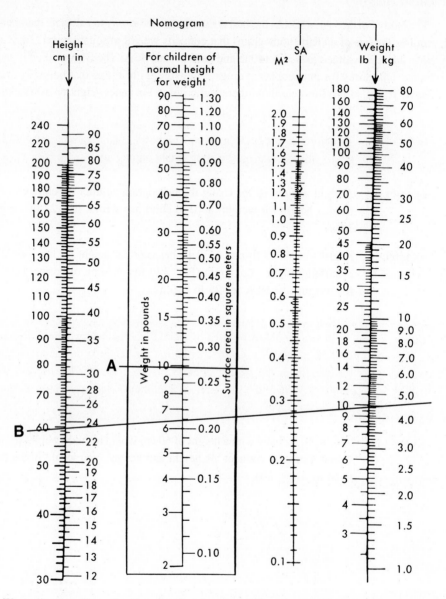

Fig. 3. West nomogram (for estimation of surface areas). **A,** When the child is normal height for weight, use the enclosed area for determining the body surface area (BSA). **B,** For a child who is under- or overweight, the surface area is indicated where a straight line connecting the height and weight intersects the surface areas (SA) column. (Nomogram modified from data of Boyd, E. by West, C.D.; from Shirkey, H.C.: Drug therapy. In Vaugn, V.C., III, and McKay, R.J., editors: Nelson's textbook of pediatrics, ed. 10, Philadelphia, 1975, W.B. Saunders Co.)

BSA Formula: $\dfrac{m^2 \text{ (child)}}{1.7 \text{ m}^2 \text{ (average adult)}} \times$ Average adult dose = Child's dose

EXAMPLE: A 10-lb child has an m^2 of 0.27, and the average adult dose of a new antibiotic is 250 mg. How many mg would be safe for the child?

$$\frac{0.27}{1.7 \text{ m}^2} \times 250 = 39.7 \text{ mg or } 40 \text{ mg}$$

EXAMPLE: A 26-lb child has an m^2 of 0.52, and the average adult dose of a tranquilizer is 15 mg. How many mg would be safe for the child?

$$\frac{0.52}{1.7 \text{ m}^2} \times 15 = 4.5 \text{ mg}$$

Steps to solving problems:

1. Check doctor's order and check recommended dose in literature.

   Ordered: 15 mg prednisone stat
   Literature: 40 mg/m² for children with Hodgkin's disease

2. Determine weight and height of child. Consult the appropriate nomogram and columns to obtain BSA in m².

   9.1 kg or 22.75 lb with normal height of 71 cm.
   BSA is approximately 0.48 m².

3. Calculate the recommended mg/m² dose in the literature using ratio and proportion (as you did with the mg/kg method), and compare it with the dose ordered for safety (recommended mg:1 m²::x mg:child's m²).

   Know   **Want to know**
   40 mg:1 m²::x mg:0.48 m²
   $x = 40 \times 0.48$
   $x = 19.20$ mg safe dose limit
   15 mg ordered
   Order is safe.

---

*Calculate kg to hundredths. Do not round.

4. If only an adult average dose is cited in the literature,* calculate the appropriate dose for the child using the BSA formula and compare it with the physician's order for safety.

$$\frac{m^2 \text{ (child)}}{1.7 \text{ (}m^2 \text{ average adult)}} \times \text{ average adult dose} = \text{ Safe dose}$$

For example, child has m^2 of 0.6 and average adult dose of a drug is 100 mg.

$$\frac{0.6}{1.7} \times 100 = 35 \text{ mg (safe dose limit)}$$

Clark's rule

$$\frac{\text{Weight of child in lb}}{150 \text{ lb}} \times \text{ Average adult dose} = \text{ Child's dose}$$

EXAMPLE: Calculate the dose of atropine sulfate for a child weighing 40 lb. Average adult dose is 0.4 mg/ml.

Weight of child: $\dfrac{40 \text{ lb}}{150 \text{ lb}} \times 0.4 \text{ mg (average adult dose)}$

$$\frac{40}{150} \times 0.4 = \frac{1.6}{15} = 0.11 \text{ mg}$$

Medication available is atropine sulfate 0.4 mg/ml.

Know	Want
0.4 mg:1 ml::0.11 mg:x ml	
0.4x = 0.11	
x = 0.27 ml†	

PROOF: $1 \times 0.11 = 0.11$
$0.4 \times 0.27 = 0.108$

---

*The literature now cites mg/kg or mg/m² for most medications for children.
†Pediatric volume less than 1 ml should be measured to hundredths in a tuberculin syringe and appropriate needle size selected.

Fried's rule

$$\frac{\text{Age in months}}{150 \text{ months}} \times \text{Average adult dose} = \text{Child's dose}$$

EXAMPLE: Calculate the dose of Valium (diazepam) for an 11-month-old baby if adult dose is 10 mg.

Age in months: $\frac{11}{150} \times 10$ mg (average adult dose)

$$\frac{11}{150} \times 10 = \frac{11\cancel{0}}{15\cancel{0}} = \frac{11}{15} = 0.733$$

Give 0.7 mg of Valium IM.

Available is Valium 10 mg/2 ml ampule. How many ml will you give?

Have   **Want**

10 mg:2 ml::0.7 mg:x ml   **PROOF:** $10 \times 0.14 = 1.4$

$10x = 1.4$ $2 \times 0.7 = 1.4$

$x = 0.14$ ml

Use a tuberculin syringe, and measure correct amount.

Young's rule

$$\frac{\text{Age of child in years}}{\text{Age of child} + 12} \times \text{Average adult dose} = \text{Child's dose}$$

EXAMPLE: Calculate the dose of IM Polycillin if adult dose is 500 mg.

$$\frac{\text{Age}}{\text{Age} + 12} = \frac{2}{2 + 12} \times 500 \text{ mg adult dose} = \frac{2}{14} \times 500 =$$

$$\frac{1}{7} \times \frac{500}{1} = \frac{500}{7} = 71 \text{ mg}$$

Available is Polycillin 500 mg per 2-ml vial. How many ml will you give?

Have   **Want**

500 mg:2 ml::71 mg:x ml   **PROOF:** $500 \times 0.28 = 140$

$500x = 142$ $2 \times 71 = 142$

$x = 0.28$ ml

1. Estimate the following weights in kg. Then convert lb to kg using the ratio and proportion method. Prove your answer.
   a. 14 lb (1 or 2 steps?)
   b. 12 lb, 2 oz (1 or 2 steps?)
   c. 10 lb
   d. 7 lb, 6 oz
   e. 15 lb, 8 oz

2. Calculate the 24-hour total dosage.
   a. 150 mg q.8h.
   b. 200 mg q.6h.
   c. 400 mcg q.4h.
   d. 50 mg t.i.d.
   e. 75 mg q.12h.

3. Calculate the safe dose ranges in mg for the following weights. Use ratio and proportion.
   a. 10 mg/kg; weight is 5 kg
   b. 5–8 mg/kg; weight is 7.3 kg
   c. 6–8 mg/kg; weight is 8 lb
   d. 3–6 mg/kg; weight is 5 lb, 8 oz
   e. 20–40 mg/kg; weight is 4 lb, 6 oz

4. State the BSA in m^2 for the following children of normal height and weight.*
   a. 4 lb
   b. 10 lb
   c. 15 lb
   d. 50 lb
   e. 70 lb

5. State the BSA in m^2 for the following children who are above or below normal height for weight.*
   a. 90 cm; 15 kg
   b. 50 cm; 11 lb
   c. 102 cm; 50 lb
   d. 50 cm; 4 kg
   e. 16 in; 7 lb

1. Doctor ordered 10 mg phenobarbital sodium IV mg q.6h. Baby's weight today is 7 lb, 2 oz. Safe range in the literature is 3 to 6 mg/kg q.24h. On hand is phenobarbital sodium injectable 65 mg/ml. What is baby's weight in kg? What is safe dosage range for this baby? Is this order safe? If so, how many ml will you prepare for each dose?

---

*Use the West nomogram (Fig. 3).
†Calculate kg to hundredths.

2. The average adult dose of Garamycin (gentamicin sulfate) is 60 mg IM t.i.d. Use the BSA chart to determine how many mg would be safe to administer to a child who weighs 11.4 kg. Medication available is labeled 80 mg/2-ml vial. If safe, how many ml would you use?*

3. Ordered: Garamycin IM 4 mg/kg/day divided into three doses. The child weighs 30 lb. The average adult dose is 60 mg q.8h. Use the BSA formula to determine the safe individual dosage for this child. Is the doctor's order safe? If so, how many mg will the child receive in 24 hours? How many ml would the child receive in each dosage? On hand is 10 mg/ml Garamycin Pediatric Injectable.*

4. Doctor ordered ampicillin 50 mg q.8h. IM. Baby weighs 5 lb, 10 oz today. Safe range for babies weighing less than 20 kg is 50 mg/kg in divided doses for 24 hours. Determine baby's weight in kg. Use the mg/kg rule to determine the safe dosage range (mg/kg) for this baby. If order is safe, calculate the correct dosage. On hand is 125 mg/5 ml ampicillin oral suspension, USP.

5. Doctor ordered Lincocin 40 mg IM b.i.d. Child weighs 9 lb, 2 oz today. Safe range for this drug is 20 mg/kg q.12h. IM. Use mg/kg method to determine if this is a safe order for the baby's weight. If so, how many ml will you give? On hand is lincomycin hydrochloride 300 mg/ml.

*Refer to BSA formula.

Worksheet* (Answers on p. 185)

1. Doctor ordered Dilantin 30 mg t.i.d. p.o. for a 2-year-old child weighing 30 lb today. Safe range for this age group is 5 mg/kg/day. Use the mg/kg method to determine if this order is safe for this child. If so, how many ml will you give? On hand is Dilantin Pediatric Suspension 125 mg/5 ml.

2. Doctor ordered ampicillin 200 mg p.o. q.6h. for a baby who weighs 12 lb, 4 oz today. Safe pediatric dosage is 100 to 200 mg/kg in divided doses for 24 hours. Is this order safe? Use mg/kg method. If safe, how many ml would you give? On hand is 125 mg/5 ml ampicillin oral suspension, USP.

3. The average adult dose of paregoric is 8 ml p.o. Use Clark's rule to determine how many ml will be safe for a 20-lb child to receive. Round to the nearest tenth.

4. Apomorphine hydrochloride 5 mg SC is the average adult dose. Available is apomorphine hydrochloride 10 mg/2-ml ampule. Use Clark's rule to compute the safe dosage for a 30-lb child.

5. Average adult dose of codeine sulfate is 30 mg. Use the BSA formula to determine the safe dosage for a child weighing 50 lb. If the doctor ordered codeine sulfate 10 mg h.s., would it be a safe order?†

---

*Calculate kg to hundredths.
†Refer to BSA formula.

Worksheet* (Answers on p. 187)

1. Furosemide 120 mg IV was ordered for a child who weighs 48 lb today. The literature states that the therapeutic range for children is 2 to 6 mg/kg daily. What is the safe dose range for this child's weight? Will you hold and clarify or give this medication?

2. Doctor ordered meperidine 15 mg IM preoperatively for a child who weighs 20 lb, 8 oz. The safe range for children is 1 to 2.2 mg/kg IM. On hand you have a tubex with 25 mg/ml. Is the order safe for this child? If it is safe, how many ml will you give?

3. Doctor ordered prednisone 20 mg/day p.o. The child weighs 30 lb and has normal height for weight. Safe dose for children is 40 mg/m^2/day p.o. Use the BSA nomogram* to determine the m^2 for this child. Is the order safe? How many mg will you give?

4. Doctor ordered meperidine 25 mg IM preoperatively for a child who weighs 30 lb. The average adult dose is 50 to 75 mg IM. Use Clark's rule to estimate the safe dose for this child. Will you give it, or will you hold and clarify?

5. Doctor ordered dactinomycin (actinomycin D, ACT) 0.20 mg IV for a child who weighs 35 lb today. On hand you have a vial containing 0.5 mg/ml. Safe pediatric dosage is 15 μg/kg/day. Using mg/kg method, calculate the maximum safe dose for this child. If it is safe, calculate how many ml you would give.

*Refer to West nomogram (Fig. 3).

■ Children's Dosages Test   (Answers on p. 189)

Solve the following problems by using the *mg/kg* rules*:

1. The doctor ordered tetracycline 200 mg IV b.i.d. for a child who weighs 45 lb. Safe range is 10 to 20 mg/kg/day in two divided doses. On hand are 250-mg vials of sterile tetracycline hydrochloride that are to be reconstituted initially with 5 ml of sterile water for injection. What is safe dosage range for this child? Is the order safe? If so, how many ml will you withdraw from the vial?

2. The doctor ordered Keflin 250 mg IM q.6h. for a child who weighs 20 lb, 4 oz. Safe range for children is 80 to 160 mg/kg. What is the safe dosage range for this child? Is the order safe? If so, how many ml will you withdraw from the vial? On hand is a 1-g vial that can be reconstituted with 4 ml for IM use.

3. The doctor ordered Lasix 20 mg p.o. stat for a child. The safe dosage for initial therapy is 2 mg/kg. The child weighed 25 lb today. What is the safe dosage for this child's weight? Is the order safe? If so, how many ml will you give? On hand is Lasix Oral Solution 10 mg/ml.

Solve the following problems by using Clark's rule:

4. Adult dose of ampicillin is 600,000 U. How much would a child weighing 90 lb receive? Available is ampicillin 300,000 U/ml. How many ml will you give?

*Calculate kg to hundredths.

5. Adult dose of penicillin is 600,000 units. How much would a 75-lb child receive? Available is penicillin 600,000 U/2 ml. How many ml will you give?

6. The average adult dose of ASA is 650 mg. A child weighing 40 lb would require how many mg? The bottle of chewable baby aspirin reads: "Each tablet contains gr 1¼." How many tablets will you give? Use BSA formula to determine safe dose.

Solve the following pediatric problems:

7. Doctor ordered Mintezol 25 mg/kg of body weight. If the child weighs 20 kg, how many mg will you give? The bottle reads: "Each 5 ml contains 250 mg." How many ml will you give?

8. Doctor ordered gr iii Liquiprin. Bottle contains 60 mg per 1.25 ml. The dropper measures 2.5 ml. How many ml will you give?

9. On hand is a pediatric oral suspension of Veetids '250' (penicillin-V potassium). The bottle contains 10 g. Directions read: "Add 117 ml water to prepare 200 ml oral solution." Doctor ordered 1 tsp q.i.d. × 10 days. How many mg will each teaspoon contain?

10. Average dose of Kantrex (kanamycin sulfate) daily is 750 to 1000 mg. Directions read: "15 mg/kg in divided doses not to exceed 1.5 g in 1 day." The baby weighs 8 lb. How many mg of Kantrex should the baby receive?

CHAPTER 10

Basic intravenous calculations

Objectives

- *Memorize two-step formula for calculating IV flow rates.*
- *Given an order for IV solutions, calculate milliliters per hour.*
- *Given the drop factor, calculate drops per minute.*
- *Use drop factor for microdrip tubing.*
- *Determine whether to start at step 1 or step 2 of IV rate calculation.*
- *Calculate IV flow rates.*
- *Calculate infusion time.*
- *Calculate units per hour for insulin and heparin infusions.*

Explanation

There are two steps in IV calculations. The first step is to find out how many *ml per hour* the IV must infuse. The second step is to calculate the *drops per minute* needed to infuse the ml/hr.

Analyze your problem. If the doctor ordered the IV to infuse for 8 hours, you must begin at step 1 to figure the ml/hr. If the order *reads* the IV is to infuse at 75 ml/hr, start at step 2.

> **RULE:** When the total volume is given, calculate the ml/hr.

$$Step\ 1: \frac{\text{Total volume (TV)}}{\text{Total time (TT)}} = \text{ml/hr}$$

EXAMPLE: ORDERED: 2000 ml D5W (dextrose 5% in water) to be infused in 8 hours. The problem is to find out how many ml/hr the patient must receive for the 2000 ml to be infused in 8 hours.

Formula:

$$\frac{\text{Total volume (TV)}}{\text{Total time (TT)}} = \text{ml/hr}$$

$$\frac{\text{Total volume (TV)}}{\text{Total time (TT)}} = \frac{2000 \text{ ml}}{8 \text{ hr}} = \text{ml/hr}$$

$$\frac{\text{TV}}{\text{TT}} = \frac{2000}{8} = 2000 \div 8 = 250 \text{ ml/hr}$$

We now know that to get 2000 ml of fluid in 8 hours the patient must get 250 ml/hr. Now calculate how many drops are needed per *minute* to infuse 250 ml/hr.

Explanation

The drop factor is the number of drops in 1 ml (or 1 cc). The diameter of the tube where the drop enters the drip chamber varies from one manufacturer to another. The bigger the tube, the fatter the drop (Fig. 4, **A**); thus it may take only 10 gtt to make a ml. The smallest unit is the microdrop (60 gtt/ml) (Fig. 4, **B**). This is used for people who can tolerate only small amounts of fluid. Drop factors of 10, 15, and 60 (microdrip) are the most common. The drop factor is found on the IV tubing box.

RULE: When the ml/hr is given, calculate the gtt/min.

Step 2: $\dfrac{\text{Drop factor or gtt/ml (IV box)}}{\text{Time in minutes}} \times \text{Total hourly volume (V/hr)} = \text{gtt/min}$

EXAMPLE: ORDERED: D5W to infuse at 250 ml/hr. Drop factor is 10.

$$\frac{\text{Drop factor (Df)}}{\text{Time (min)}} \times \text{V/hr} \qquad \frac{10 \text{ (Df)}}{60 \text{ (min)}} \times 250 \text{ (V/hr)}$$

$$\frac{10}{60} \times \frac{250}{1} = \frac{1}{6} \times \frac{250}{1} = \frac{250}{6} = 41.6 \text{ or } 42 \text{ drops/min}$$

SUMMARY: Two-step IV flow rate calculations

Step 1: $\dfrac{TV}{TT} = ml/hr$

Step 2: $\dfrac{Df}{Min} \times V/hr = gtt/min$ Remember to reduce fraction *before* multiplying.

or

$\dfrac{D}{M} \times V = gtt/min$ DMV (Department of Motor Vehicles) may be easier to remember.

REMEMBER: Reduce the fraction $\dfrac{Df}{Min}$ or $\dfrac{D}{M}$ *before* multiplying by the volume.

Which would you rather calculate?

$\dfrac{12}{60} \times 60$ or $\dfrac{1}{5} \times 60$

The reduced fraction is easier to calculate.

■ ABBREVIATIONS FOR COMMON INTRAVENOUS SOLUTIONS ■

NS	Normal saline 0.9%
1/2 NS	Normal saline 0.45%
D/RL	Dextrose with Ringer's lactate solution
D5W or 5% D/W	Dextrose 5% in water
RL or RLS	Ringer's lactate solution (electrolytes)
Isolytes	Electrolyte solutions
D5NS	Dextrose 5% in normal saline

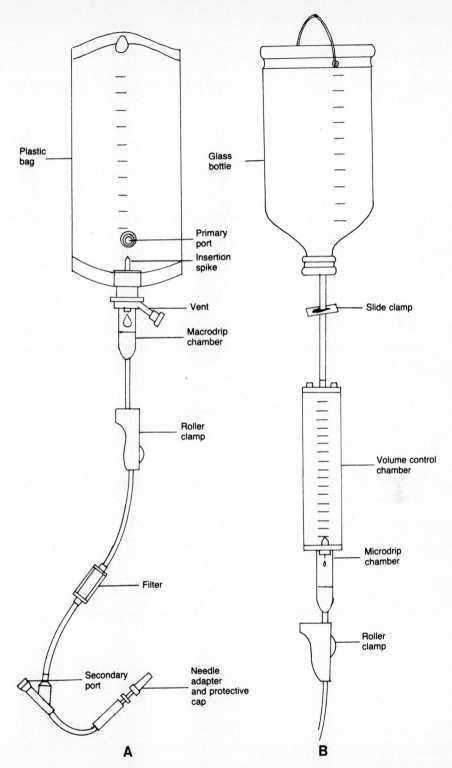

Fig. 4. Intravenous administration sets. **A,** With macrodrip chamber. **B,** With microdrip chamber. (From Clayton, B.D., et al.: Squire's basic pharmacology for nurses, ed. 8, St. Louis, 1985, The C.V. Mosby Co.)

1. Ordered: 1000 ml to be infused in 8 hours. How many gtt/min if the drop factor is 10?
   Start at step _____.

2. Ordered: 200 ml to be infused in an hour. If drop factor is 12, how many gtt/min?
   Start at step _____.

3. Ordered: 100 ml to be infused in 30 minutes. How many gtt/min if drop factor is 10?
   Start at step _____.

4. Ordered: 1500 ml to be infused in 12 hours. If drop factor is 15, how many gtt/min?
   Start at step _____.

5. Ordered: 50 ml to be infused in an hour. How many gtt/min with microdrip?

---

*FORMULA: $\dfrac{TV}{TT}$ = ml/hr $\dfrac{D}{M} \times$ V/hr = gtt/min

6. Ordered: 1500 ml to be infused in 8 hours. How many ml/hr?
   a. How many gtt/min with drop factor of 10?

   b. How many gtt/min with drop factor of 15?

7. Ordered: 75 ml to be infused in 45 minutes. Drop factor is 10. How many gtt/min?

8. Ordered: 250 ml to be infused in 90 minutes. Drop factor is microdrip. How many gtt/min?

9. Ordered: 150 ml to infuse in 40 minutes. Drop factor is 15 gtt/ml. How many gtt/min?

10. Ordered: 1000 ml to infuse at 150 ml/hr. Drop factor is 20. How many gtt/min?

Worksheet   (Answers on p. 191)

1. You have 2000 ml 5% D/W being infused for 24 hours. How many ml/hr?

2. You have 1500 ml NS. Drop factor is 15. Solution is to be given for an 8-hour period. How many ml/hr? How many gtt/min?

3. Solution of 3000 ml D5W is being infused for 24 hours with 1.5 g carbenicillin. Drop factor is 60 (microdrip). How many gtt/min? With which step will you begin?

4. You have 500 ml 0.45% NS infusing for 4 hours. Drop factor is 15. How many gtt/min?

5. Doctor ordered 1000 ml to be infused for 12 hours on microdrip. How many gtt/min will you regulate the flow?

6. Order calls for 100 ml gentamicin to be infused within 30 minutes. Drop factor is 12. How many gtt/min?

7. Doctor ordered 2000 ml for 24 hours. Drop factor is 15. How many gtt/min?

8. Ordered: 250 ml D5W is to be infused for 10 hours on a microdrip. How many gtt/min?

9. Doctor ordered 1500 ml of Ringer's lactate solution to run for 12 hours. How many ml/hr? Drop factor is 15. How many gtt/min?

10. Write your two-step formula again.

    Step 1

    Step 2

1. Ordered: 100 ml/hr. How many gtt/min if drop factor is 10? (Start at step 1 or step 2?)

2. Ordered: 1000 ml to be infused in 6 hours. How many gtt/min if drop factor is 15? (Start at step 1 or step 2?)

3. Ordered: 50 ml to be infused in 30 minutes. How many gtt/min if drop factor is 10? (Start at step 1 or 2?)

4. Ordered: 100 ml to be infused in 60 minutes. How many gtt/min if a microdrip is used? (Start at step 1 or step 2?)

5. Ordered: 2000 ml to be infused in 12 hours. Drop factor is 60.
   a. How many ml/hr?
   b. How many gtt/min?

6. Ordered: 100 ml to be infused in 30 minutes. Drop factor is 12. How many gtt/min?

7. Ordered: 1500 ml 0.45% NS in 24 hours. Drop factor is 10. How many gtt/min?

8. Ordered: 500 ml in 8 hours by microdrip. How many gtt/min?

9. Ordered: 1000 ml Ringer's lactate solution at 75 ml/hr. Drop factor is 15. How many gtt/ min?

10. Ordered: D5W continuous infusion at 85 ml/hr. Drop factor is 20. How many gtt/min?

1. Doctor ordered Keflin 4 g in 100 ml IVPB to be infused over 1 hour. The drop factor is 15.
   - How many gtt/min?

2. Order calls for ampicillin 500 mg in 50 ml IVPB to be infused in 20 minutes.
   - How many gtt/min if drop factor is 15?

3. Doctor ordered gentamicin 80 mg in 50 ml IVPB to be infused in 30 minutes.
   - How many gtt/min if drop factor is 60?

4. Order calls for Aq. penicillin 600,000 U in 100 ml IVPB to be infused in 1 hour. The drop factor is 12.
   - How many gtt/min?

5. Ordered: 250 ml NS to be infused at 60 gtt/min. The drop factor is 20 gtt/ml.
   - How long will it take to infuse?

6. Ordered: 2000 ml D5W to be infused at 40 gtt/min. The drop factor is 15 gtt/ml.
   - How long will it take to infuse?

7. Ordered: Kantrex 300 mg in 150 ml IVPB. Label reads to infuse in 40 to 60 minutes. Drop factor is microdrip.
   - How many gtt/min to infuse in 40 minutes?
   - What is the slowest infusion rate?

8. Ordered: 1000 ml 0.9% saline to infuse at 40 gtt/min. Drop factor is 15 gtt/ml.
   - How long will it take to infuse?

9. Ordered: 100 ml with 1 g Cephalin to infuse in 30 minutes by microdrip.
   - What is the gtt rate per minute?

10. Ordered: 200 ml to infuse at 50 gtt/min. Drop factor is microdrip.
    - How long will it take to infuse?

Definition

Hyperalimentation or total parenteral nutrition (TPN) is the intravenous delivery of nourishment. Protein, carbohydrates, trace minerals, vitamins, and electrolytes are delivered in individualized amounts. The carbohydrates are delivered in the form of glucose (D50W, D40W).

Hyperalimentation (TPN)   40 ml/hr =   960/24 hr
                                                     80 ml/hr = 1920/24 hr
                                                   125 ml/hr =   3000/24 hr

1. Ordered: TPN 1000 ml to be infused at 40 ml/hr. Drop factor is 20.
   - How many gtt/min?

2. Ordered: TPN 1000 ml to be infused at 80 ml/hr continuous infusion. Drop factor is 15.
   - How many ml/24 hr?
   - How many gtt/min?

3. Ordered: TPN 1000 ml to be infused at 125 ml/hr continuous infusion. Drop factor is micro-drip.
   - How many ml/hr?
   - How many gtt/min?

4. Ordered: TPN 3000 ml in 24 hr. Drop factor is 60.
   - How many gtt/min?

5. Ordered: TPN 2000 ml continuous drip in 24 hr. Drop factor is 20.
   - How many ml/hr?
   - How many gtt/min?

1. Ordered: Pitocin 125 ml/hr. You have 1000 ml RLS with 10 U of Pitocin.
   - How many hours will it take to infuse?
   - How many U/hr will be infused?

2. Ordered: Pitocin 150 ml/hr. Pharmacy has sent 1000 ml RLS with 20 U of Pitocin.
   - How many hours will it take to infuse?
   - How many U/hr will be infused?

3. Ordered: magnesium sulfate 2 g/hr. You have $MgSO_4$ 40 g/1000 ml. Microdrip.
   - How many ml/hr will deliver 2 g/hr?
   - How many gtt/min?
   - How many hours will it take to infuse?

4. Ordered: magnesium sulfate 25 ml/hr. Pharmacy has sent 1000 ml RLS with 20 g of magnesium sulfate. IMED pump-microdrip.
   - How many g/hr will infuse?
   - How many gtt/min will infuse?
   - How long will the IV infuse?

5. Ordered: magnesium sulfate 3 g/hr. Pharmacy has sent 1000 ml RLS with 40 g $MgSO_4$.
   - How many ml/hr will infuse?
   - How many gtt/min will infuse?
   - How long will the IV infuse?

Explanation

During acute phases of illness, insulin or heparin is given by the intravenous route to ensure a controlled supply of medication that will vary depending on laboratory monitoring. Infusion is usually administered with an IMED or IV pump (microdrip). To prevent insulin from being absorbed by the plastic infusion bag, albumin may be added.

> **RULE:** Begin the problem with known amount of medication in the total solution.

EXAMPLE: ORDERED: Regular insulin* 10 U/hr IV drip. Pharmacy has delivered 1000 ml 0.9% NS with 500 U regular insulin.

- How many ml/hr will infuse 10 U/hr?
- How many hours will the IV infuse?
- How many gtt/min will infuse 10 U/hr?

Have	Want to know
500 U:1000 ml::10 U:x ml	

Step 1: $500x = 1000 \times 10 = 10,000$

$500x = 10,000$

$x = 20$ ml/hr $= 10$ U of insulin

PROOF: $500 \times 20 = 10,000$
$1000 \times 10 = 10,000$

Know	Want to know
20 ml:1 hr::1000 ml:x hr	

Step 2: $20x = 1000$

$x = 50$ hr to infuse 500 U regular insulin

PROOF: $20 \times 50 = 1000$
$1 \times 1000 = 1000$

Step 3: $\dfrac{D}{M} \times V/hr = gtt/min$

$$\frac{\overset{1}{\cancel{60}}}{\underset{1}{\cancel{60}}} \times 20 = 20 \text{ gtt/min}$$

---

*Only regular insulin can be used intravenously.

1. Ordered: heparin sodium 1000 U/hr IV. Pharmacy has sent 1 L of 0.9% saline with 20,000 U of heparin.
   - How many ml/hr will deliver 1000 U?
   - How many gtt/min to infuse the ordered amount?

2. Ordered: heparin sodium 20,000 U IV in 12 hours. Pharmacy has sent 1000 ml with 20,000 U heparin sodium.
   - How many ml/hr should the IV infuse?
   - How many gtt/min will you regulate the IV?
   - How many units/hr will infuse?

3. Ordered: heparin 1500 U/hr IV. Pharmacy has sent 1 L 0.9% saline with 20,000 U of heparin.
   - How many ml/hr will deliver 1500 U?
   - How many gtt/min will infuse 1500 U/hr?
   - How many hours will the IV infuse?

4. Ordered: heparin 10,000 U in 15 hours. Pharmacy has sent 1000 ml NS with 10,000 U of heparin.
   - How many units/hr will the patient receive?
   - How many ml/hr will be infused?
   - How many gtt/min will you regulate the IV?

5. Ordered: heparin 1200 U/hr. Pharmacy has sent 500 ml NS with 10,000 U of heparin.
   - How many ml/hr will infuse 1200 U/hr?
   - How many gtt/min will you regulate the IV?

6. Ordered: 10 U/hr regular insulin IV. Pharmacy sent 500 ml 0.9% saline with 250 units regular insulin.
   - How many hours will the IV infuse?
   - How many gtt/min will deliver 10 U/hr?

7. Ordered: 6 U/hr regular insulin. You have a 10-ml vial of U 100 insulin and 250 ml of 0.9% saline. You add 100 U of regular insulin (1 ml).
   - How many ml of insulin will infuse 6 U of insulin?
   - How many gtt/min will infuse 6 U/hr?
   - How many hours will the infusion last?

8. Ordered: 8 U/hr regular insulin IV. Pharmacy has sent 250 ml NS with 100 U insulin.
   - How many ml/hr will infuse?
   - How many gtt/min will give 8 U/hr?
   - How many hours will the IV infuse?

9. Ordered: 7 U/hr regular insulin IV. Pharmacy has sent 200 ml NS with 100 U regular insulin.
   - How many ml/hr will infuse 7 U/hr?
   - How many gtt/min will deliver 7 U/hr?
   - How many hours will the IV infuse?

10. Ordered: regular insulin 9 U/hr IV. Pharmacy sent 500 ml NS with 100 U insulin.
    - How many ml/hr will infuse 9 U/hr?
    - How many gtt/min will infuse 9 U/hr?
    - How many hours will the IV infuse?

CHAPTER 10

■ Basic Intravenous Calculations Test   (Answers on p. 201)

Write the two rules or two steps *first* and then analyze your problems. Will you begin with step 1 or step 2?

1. Doctor ordered 3000 ml for 24 hours. Drop factor is 15. How many gtt/min?

2. Ordered: 75 ml to be infused in 45 minutes. Drop factor is 10. How many gtt/min?

3. Doctor ordered 1000 ml to be infused in 12 hours IV. How many gtt/min if drop factor is 12?

4. Ordered: 1200 ml to be infused in 8 hours. Drop factor is microdrip. How many gtt/min?

5. You have 2000 ml 5% D/W being infused for 24 hours. Drop factor is 10. How many gtt/min?

6. You have 1500 ml NS to infuse. Drop factor is 15. Solution is to be given over a 12-hour period. How many ml/hr? How many gtt/min?

7. You have 3000 ml 5 D/W being infused for 24 hours with 0.5 g of penicillin in each 1000 ml. Drop factor is 60, by microdrip. How many gtt/min?

8. You have 500 ml NS being infused for 6 hours. Drop factor is 13. How many gtt/min?

9. Ordered: 1000 ml to run for 12 hours on microdrip. How many gtt/min will you regulate flow?

10. Ordered: 250 ml to infuse in 90 minutes. How many gtt/min using microdrip?

CHAPTER 11

Intravenous titrations

Objectives

- *Solve titration problems by sequencing steps and using deductive reasoning.*
- *Titrate mg/kg, µg/kg, mg/min, and calculate flow rate and administration time.*

Explanation

Titration is used to administer calculated doses of potent drugs, such as dopamine or lidocaine, in IV solution. Doses are adjusted by flow according to the patient's condition. For example, 5 mg/kg/min as the initial dosage may be adjusted to deliver only 2 mg/kg/min as the patient's condition improves.

Intravenous medications are titrated according to body weight and the recommended dosage provided by the manufacturer. Critical care units and emergency departments are most likely to use this method to calculate the exact rate of flow. Because of the need to control the rate of flow carefully, medications are usually delivered through an IV machine by piggyback (IVPB), volutrol or buritrol, and direct IV push or bolus. These medications act rapidly and must be monitored for accurate delivery rate. The progress of the patient should be monitored to assess the action of the medication.

> **RULE:** The delivery rate is the final step in titrating medications. Microdrip equals 60 gtt/ml. Ml/hr and gtt/min will be the same when using microdrip.

Steps

1. Convert lb to kg. Calculate to tenths only for adults—do not round off.

2. Convert dosage symbol from insert directions (8 μg/kg/min) to the on-hand medication dosage symbol (mg). Both symbols must be the same.

3. Calculate how many mg or μg*/min are needed for the total kg of body weight.

4. Calculate total hours or minutes needed to infuse the total amount of medication.

5. Calculate total ml of medication needed.

6. Calculate gtt/min (microdrip) or ml/hr.

> **EXAMPLE:** ORDERED: 200 mg Intropin (dopamine HCl) IV drip. Directions read: "8 μg/kg/min starting with 200 mg dissolved in 250 ml 5% D/W." On hand is a 5-ml vial containing 400 mg Intropin. The patient weighs 210 lb. Current IV is infusing at 100 ml/hr (microdrip).
>
> - What will the infusion rate be?
> - Will you have to change the IV rate?
> - How long will the IV infuse?†

Steps

1. Convert lb to kg. (Calculate to tenths.)

2. Convert μg (or mcg) to what the label reads (mg).

3. Calculate mg/kg/min needed.

4. Calculate minutes/dose.

5. Calculate ml of medication ordered.

6. Calculate gtt/min.

---

*The abbreviations μg and mcg are used interchangeably.
†Plan your time to return IV to original rate.

ANSWERS

Convert lb to kg.

Step 1: 1 kg:2.2 lb::x kg:210 lb   PROOF: 2.2 × 95.4 = 209.8
       2.2x = 210   1 × 210 = 210
       x = 95.4 kg

Convert μg to mg.

Step 2: 1 mg:1000 μg::x mg:8 μg   PROOF: 1000 × 0.008 = 8
       1000x = 8   1 × 8 = 8
       x = 0.008 mg

Calculate mg/kg/min.

Step 3: 0.008 mg:1 kg::x mg:95.4 kg   PROOF: 1 × 0.76 = 0.76
       x = 0.008 × 95.4 = 0.76   0.008 × 95.4 = 0.76
       x = 0.76 mg/min for a 95.4 kg person

Calculate min/ordered dose.

Step 4: 0.76 mg:1 min::200 mg:x min   PROOF: 0.76 × 263 = 199
       0.76x = 200   1 × 200 = 200
       x = 263 min ÷ 60 = 4 hr and 23 min

Calculate ml of medication ordered.

Step 5: 5 ml:400 mg::x ml:200 mg   PROOF: 400 × 2.5 = 1000
       400x = 5 × 200 = 1000   5 × 200 = 1000
       400x = 1000
       x = 2.5 ml Intropin

Calculate gtt/min.

Step 6: $\dfrac{60}{263} \times 250 = \dfrac{15000}{263} = 57$ gtt/min

Current IV rate is 100 ml/hr = 100 gtt/min (microdrip).
Decrease IV rate to infuse 57 gtt/min.

Worksheet   (Answers on p. 201)

Convert lb to kg. Estimate answers first.

1. 135 lb
2. 205 lb
3. 98 lb
4. 176 lb
5. 159 lb

Convert μg/kg/min and mg/kg/min.

6. Weight = 61.3 kg
   15 μg/kg/min
7. Weight = 93.1 kg
   10 μg/kg/min
8. Weight = 44.5 kg
   7 μg/kg/min
9. Weight = 80 kg
   0.003 mg/kg/min
10. Weight = 72.2 kg
    0.006 mg/kg/min

Calculate minutes of infusion time. Complete problems.

11. Have 200 ml with 50,000 μg medication.
    Patient can have 919 μg/minute.

    Know   **Want to know**
    919 μg:1 min::50,000 μg:x min

12. Have 150 ml with 50,000 μg medication.
    Patient can have 931 μg/min.

    Know   **Want to know**
    931 μg:1 min::50,000 μg:x min

13. Have 250 ml with 20 mg medication.
    Patient can have 311 μg medication/min.
    Convert medication symbol so both are the same.

    Know   **Want to know**
    1 mg:1000 μg::x mg:311 μg

    Know   **Want to know**
    0.311 mg:1 min::20 mg:x min

14. Have 200 ml with 20 mg medication.
    Patient can have 0.24 mg/min.

    Know   **Want to know**
    0.24 mg/min::20 mg:x min

15. Have 100 ml with 500 μg medication.
    Patient can have 0.006 mg/min.
    Convert medication symbol so both are the same.

    Know   **Want to know**
    1 mg:1000 μg::0.006 mg:x μg

    Know   **Want to know**
    6 μg:1 min::500 μg:x min

Explanation

IVPB is an acronym for intravenous piggyback (Fig. 5). When special medications are ordered intermittently, the existing IV can be bypassed by introducing the medication through a special entry or portal. Piggyback (PB) medications are infused intermittently via the existing IV line. An extension tubing with a needle attachment is inserted into the portal or entry site. The PB infusion is usually 50 to 250 ml of medicated solution.

Elevating the IVPB 12 inches above the existing IV allows the PB to infuse by gravity. When the PB is finished, the *existing* IV will resume at the rate set for the IVPB. The nurse must remember to regulate the IV to the *previous* rate.

> **RULE:** Return the IV to the original rate after the PB has been infused.

Volutrol and buritrol administer controlled amounts of medication solution (Fig. 6). The IV tubing has a special pouch or container that holds 100 ml. Medication is injected into the volutrol/buritrol via the portal. The bag or container is then filled with the existing IV solution and the main IV clamped until the medication has been infused. The medication can be controlled (gtt/min) by the regulator below the volutrol/buritrol.

11B Worksheet   (Answers on p. 203)

1. Ordered: dobutamine HCl (Dobutrex) 200 mg IV drip. Medication reads 250 mg/20 ml. Further dilute to at least 50 ml, and administer as a continuous infusion at the usual dose of 2.5 to 10 μg/kg/min. The patient weighed 155 lb today. The current IV is infusing at 125 ml/hr.
   - What will be the infusion rate (gtt/min)?
   - Will you change the existing IV rate?
   - How many minutes or hours will the IV infuse?

Steps

1. Convert lb to kg. Calculate to tenths for adults.

2. Convert medication symbol from insert (10 μg/kg/min) to the on-hand medication symbol (mg).

3. Calculate mg/min for the kg of body weight.

4. Calculate the minutes or hours it will take to infuse the total ordered dose.

5. Calculate the ml of medication ordered.

6. Calculate the gtt/min.

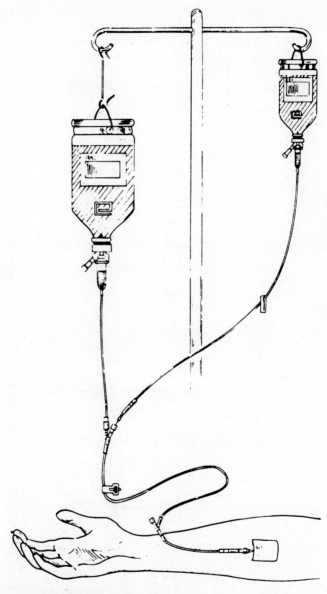

Fig. 5. Intravenous piggyback (IVPB) administration setup. Note that the smaller bottle is hung higher than the primary bottle. (From Clayton, B.D., et al: Squire's basic pharmacology for nurses, ed. 8, St. Louis, 1985, The C.V. Mosby Co.)

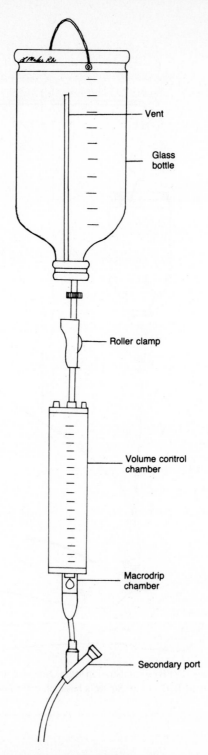

Vent

Glass
bottle

Roller clamp

Volume control
chamber

Macrodrip
chamber

Secondary port

Fig. 6. Volutrol intravenous administration set. (From Clayton, B.D., et al.: Squire's basic pharmacology for nurses, ed. 8, St. Louis, 1985, The C.V. Mosby Co.)

2. Ordered: Sodium nitroprusside (Nipride) 50 mg IV drip stat. Medication insert reads: "Usual dose is 3 μg/kg/min. Each 50 mg must be dissolved with 2 to 3 ml of D5W. Further dilute in a minimum of 250 ml of D5W for administration. Protect bottle and tubing from sunlight. A potent, rapid-acting antihypertensive." Current IV is infusing at 85 ml/hr. The patient weighs 165 lb.
   - What will be the infusion rate (gtt/min)?
   - Will you change the existing IV rate?

   Steps

   1. Convert lb to kg. Calculate to tenths for adults.

   2. Convert μg to mg.

   3. Calculate the mg/kg/min.

   4. Calculate min/ordered dose.

   5. Calculate gtt/min.

3. Ordered: lidocaine 4 mg/min IV drip for arrhythmia. Literature reads: "For continuous infusion administer at the rate of 1 to 4 mg/min (20 to 50 μg/kg/min.) To prepare IV solution, add 1 g Xylocaine HCl to 1 L of 5% D/W. 1 g in 1000 ml = 0.1% solution. Each ml will contain approximately 1 mg. No more than 200 to 300 mg should be administered during a 1-hour period. Monitor patient on ECG." Patient weighs 182 lb. Current IV rate is 100 ml/hr.
   - Is 4 mg/min a safe dose for a 1-hour period?
   - How many ml/hr will deliver 4 mg/min?
   - Will you change the IV rate?

   Steps

   1. Convert lb to kg.

   2. Calculate the safe maximum μg/kg/min.

   3. Convert μg to mg/min.

   4. Using the 4 mg/min rate, calculate the mg to be infused in 1 hour.

   5. Calculate ml/hr to be infused and gtt/min (microdrip).

4. Ordered: 150 mg Coly-Mycin M q.12h. IV volutrol. Medication directions read: "Adults, children, and infants 2.5 to 5 mg/kg of body weight/24 hr. 150 mg vial is diluted with 2 ml sterile water for injection. 1 ml equals 75 mg. Further dilute each single dose with 20 ml sterile water for injection for direct IV administration. May be further diluted with 50 ml of more D5W, NS, LRS and given through the Y connection or additive infusion tubing. Further dilute to a volume of 100 ml for use in volutrol set. Infuse in 20 to 40 minutes." Patient weighed 176 lb. IV is infusing at 150 ml/hr.
   - Is this a safe dose?
   - How many ml of medication will you use?
   - What is the infusion rate for 20 minutes and for 40 minutes?
   - Will you have to change the IV rate?

   ### Steps

   1. Convert lb to kg.

   2. Calculate safe dose.

   3. Calculate amount of medication for volutrol dilution.

   4. Calculate gtt/min for 20 and 40 minutes.

5. Ordered: Aldomet (methyldopate hydrochloride) 0.5 g q.6h. Medication insert reads: "Usual dose: 7 to 10 mg/kg every 6 hours. Up to 1 g every 6 hours. Single dose is diluted in 100 to 200 ml of 5% dextrose water and given as an infusion. Infuse each dose over 30 to 60 minutes. Incompatible with amphotericin B and tetracycline. Antidote: dopamine (Intropin) or norepinephrine (Levophed)." Patient weighs 155 lb. Pharmacy has sent 200/ml D5W with 500 mg Aldomet. Infusion set is a microdrip infusing at a rate of 100 ml/hr.
   - Is this a safe dose?
   - Will you have to change the infusion rate?

   ### Steps

   1. Convert lb to kg.

   2. Calculate safe dose.

   3. Convert order in g to mg.

   4. Calculate gtt/min.

CHAPTER 12

Solutions

Objectives

- *Calculate percent of sodium chloride in normal saline solution.*
- *Calculate percent solution problem using ratio and proportion method.**

Explanation

A solution consists of two parts: the solvent (usually water) and the solute (a solid, liquid, or gas) dissolved in the solvent. Solution problems are percent problems. Remember that *percentage* means hundred*ths*. A percent number is a fraction whose top number is stated and bottom number is understood to be 100. 20% is the same as ²⁰/₁₀₀. To make a ratio out of a fraction, put the numerator on the left and the denominator on the right. The fraction ²⁰/₁₀₀ is the same as the ratio 20:100.

One ml (or cc) of water weighs 1 g. Therefore g and ml (or cc) can be used interchangeably. If the solute (part being dissolved) is a liquid, then ml (or cc) can be used. (The use of ml is preferred over cc, because cc is properly used with gases. Nevertheless, cc is occasionally used in this text.) If the solute is a solid such as NaCl (salt) or tablets, then the g symbol is used.

Normal saline (isotonic sodium chloride) is 0.9%. As a ratio it is *always* written 0.9:100. Half-strength NaCl is 0.45%. As a ratio, it is *always* written 0.45:100.

> **RULE:** Set up a ratio and proportion with what you *have* on hand on the *left* and what you *want* to make on the *right*.

EXAMPLE: Make up 250 ml of a 20% acetic acid solution.

Have	Want

Step 1: 20 ml acetic acid:100 ml water::x ml acetic acid:250 ml water

$100x = 5000$ PROOF: $100 \times 50 = 5000$
$x = 50$ ml acetic acid for a 20% solution $20 \times 250 = 5000$

---

*Few solutions are prepared by nurses.

When working with liquids such as acetic acid, you must *subtract* the amount of *full-strength* acetic acid needed (in this problem it is 50 ml) from the total amount of solution ordered to determine how much water to add. When you have figured out how much solvent to use, pour exact amount into the container first then fill to the total amount of solution ordered.

Step 2: Use 50 ml of full-strength acetic acid. The total amount of solution ordered was 250 ml.

> 250 ml ordered
> -50 ml full-strength acetic acid
> 200 ml water added to 50 ml of 20% acetic acid = 250 ml of 20% solution

NOTE: The ratio and proportion setup works when a solution is prepared from a *full-strength* solid or liquid such as salt or 100% solutions.

RULE:	If the solution you are to use for the preparation of the desired solution is a ratio, just use the ratio for the *have* side or *left* side of the equation.

EXAMPLE: Make up 1 pint of a 1:1000 Zephiran chloride solution.

> **Have**   **Want**
>
> *Step 1:* 1 g:1000 ml::x g:500 ml
> $1000x = 500$
> $x = 0.5$ g

> *Step 2:* You will measure ½ g or ml of 1:1000 Zephiran chloride solution and pour it into 499.5 ml of water = 500 ml of 1:1000 solution.

NOTE: When the answer is in grams and the tablets are in grains, you must set up a ratio and proportion; 1 g = gr 15.

12A Worksheet   (Answers on p. 207)

1. Make up 500 ml of normal saline solution. How many g of salt will you use? How many tsp is this?

2. Make up 200 ml of 1:1 ½ strength saline and peroxide. Irrigate wound t.i.d. with 60 ml normal saline solution. How many g or tsp of salt will you add?

3. Ordered: 300 ml of a 5% acetic acid solution. How much full-strength acetic acid will you use and how much water?

4. Ordered: 250 ml of a 10% acetic acid solution. How much full-strength acetic acid will you use and how much water?

5. Ordered: 150 ml of normal saline solution for a mouthwash. How much salt will you use? How can this problem be simplified?

6. Make up 200 ml of a 10% solution of acetic acid from full-strength liquid. How many ml of acetic acid will you use?

7. Prepare NS solution (0.9%) as an enema. You will use _____ tsp of table salt in 1000 ml of H_2O.

8. Prepare an NS throat irrigation. You will mix _____ tsp of salt with 500 ml H_2O.

9. You are to give 1½% vinegar douche. The douche bag holds 1 qt. You will add _____ tsp of vinegar to 1 qt of H$_2$O.

10. Prepare 500 ml of a 40% Betadine solution using NS.

CHAPTER 12

■ Solutions Test   (Answers on p. 210)

1. Prepare 4 L of a 1:500 ml solution of Lysol. How many ml of Lysol will you need?

2. Prepare 250 ml of a 50% solution of betadine and ½ NS.

3. Prepare 1 L of a 1:750 solution of potassium permanganate. How many g of KMnO$_4$ will you need?

4. Prepare 1 pt of a 1:750 solution of potassium permanganate. Tablets of KMnO$_4$ containing gr 1 each are in stock. How many grains or tablets will you use? Is this a one-step or a two-step problem?

5. Prepare 300 ml of a 30% peroxide solution using 0.9% NS.

Comprehensive examination (Answers on p. 210)

Show work, label answers, and prove:

1. Doctor has ordered elix. of phenobarbital 0.5 g p.o. a.c. t.i.d. The label reads elix. of phenobarb. 250 mg/ml. How many ml for each dose? How many per day?

2. Doctor orders quinidine 200 mg IM. On hand is a vial labeled quinidine 0.1 g/3 ml. How many ml will you give?

3. Doctor orders 500 mg of Diuril. On hand are 0.25 g tablets. How many tablets will you give?

4. You are to give atropine gr $\frac{1}{200}$. On hand is a vial labeled gr $\frac{1}{150}$ in 0.5 cc. How many ml will you give?

5. You are to give 200,000 units of penicillin. On hand is a multiple-dose vial labeled 1,000,000 U in 10 cc. How many ml will you give?

6. A patient is to receive 500 ml of NS intravenously in 8 hours. How many ml/hr should the patient receive?

7. The above as an IV dose should be infused at _____ gtt/min. Drop factor is 15.

8. The patient is to receive 1000 ml of D5W in 8 hr. How many ml/hr will that be?

9. An IV fluid is being infused at a rate of 100 ml/hr. This should run at _____ gtt/min. Drop factor is 10 gtt/ml.

10. Doctor ordered penicillin 300,000 units. On hand is a penicillin 5-ml vial stating: "Add 5 ml sterile H_2O to make penicillin 600,000 U/2 ml." How many ml will you give?

11. You are to give penicillin 1.3 million units stat. On hand is a vial labeled 10,000,000 units in 10 ml. You will give _____ ml.

12. Ordered: penicillin 600,000 units IM q.8h. Available: penicillin 2,000,000 units per 5 ml. You will give _____ ml every 8 hours.

13. Ordered is codeine gr ⅙. On hand is gr ¼ per ml. How many ml will you give?

14. On hand: codeine (tablets) gr ½ p.o. Ordered: 60 mg. How many tablets will you give?

15. Ordered: digoxin 0.125 mg. On hand is an ampule labeled digoxin 0.25 mg/ml. How many ml will you give?

16. Doctor ordered 24 units of U 100 every AM ½ hr a.c. regular insulin. You are out of insulin syringes. How many ml will you give in a tuberculin syringe?

17. Ordered: atropine gr ½₀₀. On hand is atropine gr ⅟₁₅₀ per 0.5 cc. How many minims will you give?

18. Ordered: heparin sodium 5000 U stat. On hand you have a vial labeled heparin sodium 20,000 U per ml. How many ml will you give (nearest hundredth)?

19. Ordered: 75 mg meperidine and Vistaril 25 mg on call to the O.R. Have: Demerol 100 mg/ml in a prefilled tube and a 2 ml vial of Vistaril containing 100 mg. How many total ml will you prepare? (Round off to tenths.)

20. Ordered: atropine sulfate gr $\frac{1}{150}$. The pharmacist has sent atropine sulfate 0.43 mg/0.5 ml. How many ml will you give?

21. Prepare a normal saline solution (0.9%) as a gargle for a sore throat. You will use _____ tsp of table salt per pint of water.

22. Doctor ordered aminophylline suppository 0.5 g. On hand you have aminophylline suppository gr viiss. How many will you give?

23. Make up 500 ml of a 20% acetic acid solution.

24. Doctor ordered ℥ ss of elixir of terpin hydrate with codeine. How many ml will you give? How many teaspoons is this?

25. Ordered: thyroid tablets 120 mg daily AM. On hand are tablets labeled thyroid gr i. How many tablets or what part of a tablet will you give?

26. Your weight is 55 kg. This is equivalent to how many pounds? (Estimate first.)

27. Doctor ordered prednisone 50 mg for a child of normal height who weighs 60 lb. The literature recommends 40 mg/m². Will you give or hold and clarify the order? Show all work.

28. Doctor ordered tetracycline 100 mg IV b.i.d. for a child who weighs 15 lb, 8 oz. Safe range is 10 to 20 mg/kg/day in two divided doses. On hand are 250-mg vials of sterile tetracycline hydrochloride that are to be reconstituted initially with 5 ml of sterile water for injection. What is the safe dosage range for this child? Is the order safe? If so, how many ml will you withdraw from the vial?

29. Ordered: insulin 8 U/hr IV. Pharmacy has sent 250 ml NS with 50 units regular insulin. How many drops per minute will give you 8 U/hr using microdrip tubing?

30. Ordered: heparin 500 U/hr IV. Pharmacy has sent 500 ml of D5W with 10,000 units of heparin sodium. How many drops per minute will be needed to infuse 500 U/hr? (Use microdrip.)

Answers

1. 6¼
2. 5⅟₇
3. ³⁸/₉
4. ¹⁹/₂
5. 66
6. 45
7. 1¹/₃₀
8. 6¹⁹/₂₄
9. ¹³/₂₈
10. 4⅞
11. ¹/₁₂
12. ⅓ or ⁸/₂₄
13. ⅚
14. ¹⁸/₄₀ or ⁹/₂₀
15. ¹/₅₀
16. ⁴/₁₉
17. .14
18. 3.016

19. 4.905
20. 28.708
21. 2.96
22. 0.8241
23. 0.0036
24. 1.5
25. 10.055
26. 98.095
27. 0.534
28. 9.125
29. 9.45
30. 73.675
31. ⁷/₁₀
32. ¹²³/₂₅₀
33. 0.17 and ¹⁷/₁₀₀
34. 0.125 and 12.5%
35. ¹⁴/₁₀₀₀ and 1.4%

General mathematics review

☐ 1A   (p. 4)

1. 1
2. $3\frac{1}{4}$
3. 3
4. $1\frac{5}{9}$
5. $5\frac{2}{3}$
6. 4
7. $1\frac{3}{4}$
8. $1\frac{7}{8}$
9. 3
10. $6\frac{5}{6}$

☐ 1B   (p. 5)

1. $\frac{6}{5}$
2. $\frac{5}{4}$
3. $\frac{49}{3}$
4. $\frac{43}{12}$
5. $\frac{68}{5}$
6. $\frac{35}{8}$
7. $\frac{23}{6}$
8. $\frac{21}{8}$
9. $\frac{63}{6}$
10. $\frac{377}{3}$

☐ 1C   (p. 7)

1.
$$\begin{array}{r} \frac{1}{5} \\ +\frac{2}{5} \\ \hline \frac{3}{5} \end{array}$$

2.
$$\begin{array}{r} \frac{3}{5} = \frac{9}{15} \\ +\frac{2}{3} = \frac{10}{15} \\ \hline \frac{19}{15} = 1\frac{4}{15} \end{array}$$

3.
$$\begin{array}{r} 6\frac{1}{6} = 6\frac{4}{24} \\ +9\frac{5}{8} = 9\frac{15}{24} \\ \hline 15\frac{19}{24} \end{array}$$

4.
$$\begin{array}{r} 1\frac{3}{8} = 1\frac{15}{40} \\ +9\frac{9}{10} = 9\frac{36}{40} \\ \hline 10\frac{51}{40} = 11\frac{11}{40} \end{array}$$

5.
$$\begin{array}{r} 2\frac{1}{4} = 2\frac{2}{8} \\ +3\frac{1}{8} = 3\frac{1}{8} \\ \hline 5\frac{3}{8} \end{array}$$

6.
$$\begin{array}{r} \frac{1}{8} = \frac{9}{72} \\ \frac{1}{4} = \frac{18}{72} \\ +\frac{2}{9} = \frac{16}{72} \\ \hline \frac{43}{72} \end{array}$$

7.
$$\begin{array}{r} \frac{7}{9} = \frac{70}{90} \\ \frac{4}{5} = \frac{72}{90} \\ +\frac{9}{10} = \frac{81}{90} \\ \hline \frac{223}{90} = 2\frac{43}{90} \end{array}$$

8.
$$\begin{array}{r} 3\frac{1}{4} \\ +9\frac{3}{4} \\ \hline 12\frac{4}{4} = 13 \end{array}$$

9.
$$\begin{array}{r} 8\frac{2}{5} = 8\frac{4}{10} \\ 14\frac{7}{10} = 14\frac{7}{10} \\ + 9\frac{9}{10} = 9\frac{9}{10} \\ \hline 31\frac{20}{10} = 33 \end{array}$$

10.
$$\begin{array}{r} 2\frac{1}{3} = 2\frac{2}{6} \\ 4\frac{1}{6} = 4\frac{1}{6} \\ \hline 6\frac{3}{6} = 6\frac{1}{2} \end{array}$$

□ **1D** (p. 9)

1. $\frac{4}{5} = \frac{8}{10}$

    $\underline{-\frac{1}{2} = \frac{5}{10}}$

           $\frac{3}{10}$

2. $7\frac{16}{24} = 7\frac{16}{24}$

    $\underline{-3\frac{1}{8} = 3\frac{3}{24}}$

           $4\frac{13}{24}$

3. $21\frac{7}{16} = 20\frac{23}{16}$ Must borrow from whole number.

    $\underline{-\ \ 7\frac{12}{16} = \ \ 7\frac{12}{16}}$

           $13\frac{11}{16}$

4. $\frac{27}{32}$

    $\underline{-\frac{18}{32}}$

      $\frac{9}{32}$

5. $6\frac{3}{10} = 6\frac{3}{10}$

    $\underline{-2\frac{1}{5} = 2\frac{2}{10}}$

          $4\frac{1}{10}$

6. $\frac{7}{8} = \frac{21}{24}$

    $\underline{-\frac{2}{3} = \frac{16}{24}}$

        $\frac{5}{24}$

7. $3\frac{5}{8}$

    $\underline{-1\frac{3}{8}}$

    $2\frac{2}{8} = 2\frac{1}{4}$

8. $5\frac{3}{7} = 4\frac{10}{7}$ Must borrow from whole number.

    $\underline{-1\frac{6}{7} = 1\frac{6}{7}}$

         $3\frac{4}{7}$

9. $7\ \ = 6\frac{4}{4}$ Must borrow from whole number.

    $\underline{-1\frac{3}{4} = 1\frac{3}{4}}$

         $5\frac{1}{4}$

10. $2\frac{7}{8} = 2\frac{7}{8}$

    $\underline{-\ \frac{3}{4} = -\frac{6}{8}}$

          $2\frac{1}{8}$

1. $\frac{1}{3} \times \frac{2}{4} = \frac{2}{12} = \frac{1}{6}$

2. $5\frac{1}{2} \times 3\frac{1}{8} = \frac{11}{2} \times \frac{25}{8} = \frac{275}{16} = 275 \div 16 = 17\frac{3}{16}$

3. $1\frac{3}{4} \times 3\frac{1}{7} = \frac{\overset{1}{\cancel{7}}}{4} \times \frac{22}{\underset{1}{\cancel{7}}} = \frac{22}{4} = 22 \div 4 = 5\frac{1}{2}$

4. $4 \times 3\frac{1}{8} = 4 \times \frac{25}{8} = \frac{100}{8} = 12\frac{1}{2}$

5. $\frac{2}{4} \times 2\frac{1}{6} = \frac{\overset{1}{\cancel{2}}}{4} \times \frac{13}{\underset{3}{\cancel{6}}} = \frac{13}{12} = 1\frac{1}{12}$

6. $\frac{1}{5} \times \frac{1}{3} = \frac{1}{15}$

7. $\frac{3}{4} \times \frac{5}{8} = \frac{15}{32}$

8. $\frac{5}{6} \times 1\frac{9}{16} = \frac{5}{6} \times \frac{25}{16} = \frac{125}{96} = 125 \div 96 = 1\frac{29}{96}$

9. $\frac{5}{100} \times 900 = \frac{5}{\underset{1}{\cancel{100}}} \times \frac{\overset{9}{\cancel{900}}}{1} = 45$

10. $2\frac{1}{10} \times 4\frac{1}{3} = \frac{\overset{7}{\cancel{21}}}{10} \times \frac{13}{\underset{1}{\cancel{3}}} = \frac{91}{10} = 9\frac{1}{10}$

1. $\frac{2}{5} \div \frac{5}{8} = \frac{2}{5} \times \frac{8}{5} = \frac{16}{25}$

2. $8\frac{3}{4} \div 15 = \frac{\overset{7}{\cancel{35}}}{4} \times \frac{1}{\underset{3}{\cancel{15}}} = \frac{7}{12}$

3. $\frac{3}{4} \div \frac{1}{8} = \frac{3}{\underset{1}{\cancel{4}}} \times \frac{\overset{2}{\cancel{8}}}{1} = 6$

4. $\frac{1}{16} \div \frac{1}{4} = \frac{1}{\underset{4}{\cancel{16}}} \times \frac{\overset{1}{\cancel{4}}}{1} = \frac{1}{4}$

5. $\frac{1}{3} \div \frac{1}{2} = \frac{1}{3} \times \frac{2}{1} = \frac{2}{3}$

6. $\frac{3}{4} \div 6 = \frac{\overset{1}{\cancel{3}}}{4} \times \frac{1}{\underset{2}{\cancel{6}}} = \frac{1}{8}$

7. $2 \div \frac{1}{5} = \frac{2}{1} \times \frac{5}{1} = 10$

8. $3\frac{3}{8} \div 4\frac{1}{2} = \frac{27}{8} \div \frac{9}{2} = \frac{\overset{3}{\cancel{27}}}{\underset{4}{\cancel{8}}} \times \frac{\overset{1}{\cancel{2}}}{\underset{1}{\cancel{9}}} = \frac{3}{4}$

9. $\frac{3}{5} \div \frac{3}{8} = \frac{\overset{1}{\cancel{3}}}{5} \times \frac{8}{\underset{1}{\cancel{3}}} = \frac{8}{5} = 1\frac{3}{5}$

10. $4 \div 2\frac{1}{8} = \frac{4}{1} \times \frac{8}{17} = \frac{32}{17} = 1\frac{15}{17}$

□ **1G**   (p. 12)

1. ⅓
2. ⅟₁₅₀
3. ⅟₂₅₀
4. ⅛
5. More
6. Less
7. Less
8. Less
9. More
10. Less

□ **1H**   (p. 15)

1. Eight hundredths
2. Ninety-two thousandths
3. Seventeen ten-thousandths
4. Three thousand two hundred eighty-seven and four hundred sixty-seven thousandths
5. Six ten-thousandths
6. One hundred and one hundredth
7. 0.36
8. 0.003
9. 0.0008
10. 2.017
11. 0.05
12. 4.1
13. 24.2
14. 15.01
15. 9.0002
16. 3.008
17. 100.018
18. 18.15
19. 0.055
20. 34.1

```
          3.3
1.  48)158.4
        144
         14 4
         14 4
```

```
           3 3.333
2.  6.0̬)200̬0̬000
        180
         20 0
         18 0
          2 0 0
          1 8 0
            2 00
            1 80
              200
              180
```

```
          2.51
3.  6)15.06
       12
        30
        30
         6
         6
```

```
            91.264
4.  0.87̬)79.40̬000
         78 3̬
          1 10
            87
           23 0
           17 4
            5 60
            5 22
              380
              348
```

```
             8 60.
5.  0.78̬)670.80̬
         624̬
          46 8
          46 8
```

```
            32.345
6.  2.43̬)78.60̬000
         72 9
          5 70
          4 86
            84 0
            72 9
            11 10
             9 72
             1 380
             1 215
```

```
             3.265
7.  8.2̬)26.7̬800
        24 6
         2 1 8
         1 6 4
           5 40
           4 92
             480
             410
```

```
             46.107
8.  5.78̬)266.50̬000
         231 2̬
          35 30
          34 68
            62 0
            57 8
             4 200
             4 046
```

```
            1.661
9.  6.5̬)10.8̬000
        6 5
        4 30
        3 90
         4 00
         3 90
          100
           65
```

```
           7.653
10.  10)76.530
        70
        6 5
        6 0
         53
         50
          30
          30
```

□ 1J   (p. 18)

1.   0.8
    +0.5
     1.3

2.   3.27
     0.06
    +2.
     5.33

3.   5.01
    +2.999
     8.009

4.   15.6
      0.19
    +200.
    215.79

5.   210.79
      2.
    + 68.4
    281.19

6.   88.6
     576.46
    + 79.
     744.06

7.   6.77
     102.
    + 88.3
     197.07

8.   79.4
     68.44
    + 3.
    150.84

9.   10.56
    +356.4
    366.96

10.   99.7
     +293.23
      392.93

□ 1K   (p. 19)

1.   3.14   You do not have to multiply zeros. Count 5 places in from the right, adding zeros where
     ×0.002   needed.
     0.00628

2.   95.26   Count 5 decimal places in from the right.
     ×1.125
     47630
     19052
      9526
      9526
    107.16750

3.   0.5   Count 1 decimal place in from the right.
    ×100
    50.0

4.   2.14   Count 4 decimal places in from the right, adding zeros as needed.
    ×0.03
    0.0642

5.　36.8
　×70.1
　368
2576
2579.68

7.　90.1
　×88
7208
7208
7928.8

9.　54.5
　×21
　545
1090
1144.5

6.　203.7
　×28
16296
4074
5703.6

8.　2.76
　×0.003
0.00828

10.　200
　×0.2
40.0

□ **1L**　(p. 20)

1.　98.4
　−66.50
　31.90

5.　266.44
　−0.56
265.88

9.　1.723
　−0.683
　1.040

2.　108.56
　−5.40
103.16

6.　7.066
　−0.200
　6.866

10.　0.8100
　−0.6701
　0.1399

3.　0.450
　−0.367
　0.083

7.　34.678
　−0.502
34.176

4.　21.78
　−19.88
　1.90

8.　78.567
　−6.77
71.797

□ **1M**　(p. 22)

1. $\dfrac{4\cancel{0}}{10\cancel{0}} = \dfrac{2}{5}$

5. $1\dfrac{32}{100} = 1\frac{8}{25}$

8. $\dfrac{2\cancel{0}}{10\cancel{0}} = \dfrac{1}{5}$

2. $\dfrac{8}{10} = \dfrac{4}{5}$

6. $\dfrac{50\cancel{0}}{100\cancel{0}} = \dfrac{1}{2}$

9. $\dfrac{65}{100} = \dfrac{13}{20}$

3. $\dfrac{25\cancel{0}}{100\cancel{0}} = \dfrac{1}{4}$

7. $\dfrac{75\cancel{0}}{100\cancel{0}} = \dfrac{3}{4}$

10. $\dfrac{70\cancel{0}}{100\cancel{0}} = \dfrac{7}{10}$

4. $4\dfrac{08}{100} = 4\frac{2}{25}$

□ **1N**   (p. 23)

```
              0.19
1.  100)19.00
           10 0
            9 00
            9 00


             1.285
2.  7)9.00
       7
       2 0
       1 4
         60
         56
         40
         35


3.  5⁹⁄₁₆ = 5 × 16 + 9 = ⁸⁹⁄₁₆
             5.562½
    16)89.000
        80
         9 0
         8 0
         1 00
           96
           40
           32
            8


              0.2
4.  5)1.0
       1.0


             0.666
5.  3)2.000
       1 8
         20
         18
         20
         18
```

```
             0.5
6.  2)1.0
       1.0


            0.083
7.  12)1.000
         96
         40
         36


            0.75
8.  8)6.00
       5 6
         40
         40


             0.075
9.  200)15.000
         14 00
          1 000
          1 000


            2.5
10. 8)20.0
       16
        4 0
        4 0
```

☐ 1O   (p. 25)

1. Fraction: ⅔
   Decimal: 0.67

2. Decimal: 0.5
   Percent: 50%

3. Fraction: ¹³⁄₂₀₀
   Decimal: 0.065

4. Decimal: 0.0833
   Percent: 8.33%

5. Decimal: 0.003
   Percent: 0.3%

6. Fraction: ¹⁄₁₀
   Percent: 10%

7. Fraction: ²⁵⁰⁄₁₀₀ = ⁵⁄₂
   Decimal: 2.5

8. Fraction: ⁷⁄₂₀
   Percent: 35%

9. Decimal: 0.8
   Percent: 80%

10. Fraction: ⁷⁸⁄₁₀₀ = ³⁹⁄₅₀
    Decimal: 0.78

☐ 1P   (p. 26)

1.
```
    240
  ×1.14
    960
    240
    240
 273.60
```

2.
```
  1500
  ×.02
 30.00
```

3. $\dfrac{½}{100} = \dfrac{1}{2} \div \dfrac{100}{1} = \dfrac{1}{2} \times \dfrac{1}{100} = \dfrac{1}{200} =$

```
     .005        9328
200)1.000       ×.005
              46.640    Answer
```

4. $\dfrac{⅓}{100} = \dfrac{1}{3} \div \dfrac{100}{1} = \dfrac{1}{3} \times \dfrac{1}{100} = \dfrac{1}{300} =$

```
     .003         930
300)1.000        ×.003
     900        2.790    Answer
     100
```

5.
```
    50
  ×.28
   400
   100
 14.00
```

6.
```
   200
  ×.09
 18.00
```

7.
```
    400
  ×1.20
   8000
    400
 480.00
```

8.
```
 105.80
   ×.05
 5.2900
```

9.
```
    520
   ×.10
  52.00
```

10.
```
   40.80
    ×.03
  1.2240
```

General Mathematics Test (p. 27)

1. $5\frac{4}{6} = 5\frac{2}{3}$	13. $\frac{24}{4} = 6$	25. 3.300
2. $6\frac{6}{7}$	14. $\frac{3}{4}$	26. 91.264
3. $\frac{68}{5}$	15. $\frac{1}{250}$	27. 1.1875
4. $\frac{23}{6}$	16. $\frac{2}{13}$	28. 8.0625
5. 20	17. 0.36	29. 12.48
6. 40	18. 2.017	30. 583.00
7. $\frac{19}{36}$	19. 8.009	31. $\frac{2}{5}$
8. $10\frac{7}{8}$	20. 60.97	32. $\frac{57}{200}$
9. $\frac{5}{24}$	21. 3.824	33. 0.43 and $\frac{43}{100}$
10. 1	22. 0.1562	34. 0.10 and 10%
11. $\frac{1}{15}$	23. 0.000010	35. $\frac{29}{1000}$ and 2.9%
12. $\frac{10}{48} = \frac{5}{24}$	24. 3.5	

Ratio and proportion

☐ 2A (p. 29)

1. $\frac{2}{4} = \frac{1}{2}$	5. $\frac{43}{86} = \frac{1}{2}$	8. $\frac{1}{5}$
2. $\frac{4}{6} = \frac{2}{3}$	6. $\frac{2}{13}$	9. $\frac{1}{150}$
3. $\frac{2}{500} = \frac{1}{250}$	7. $\frac{7}{49} = \frac{1}{7}$	10. $\frac{4}{100} = \frac{1}{25}$
4. $\frac{6}{1000} = \frac{3}{500}$		

☐ 2B (p. 31)

REMEMBER: Always put x on the left.

1. $\frac{1}{2}:x::1:8$
   $1x = \frac{1}{2} \times 8$
   $x = \frac{1}{2} \times \frac{8}{1} = 4$
   $x = 4$

   PROOF: $4 \times 1 = 4$
   $\frac{1}{2} \times 8 = 4$

2. $9:x::5:300$
   $5x = 9 \times 300$
   $5x = 2700$

   $\frac{\cancel{5}x}{\cancel{5}} = \frac{2700}{5} = 2700 \div 5 = 540$

   $x = 540$

   PROOF: $540 \times 5 = 2700$
   $9 \times 300 = 2700$

■ 145

3. $^1/_{1000} : ^1/_{100} :: x : 60$

   $^1/_{100}x = ^1/_{1000} \times 60$

$$\frac{1}{100x} = \frac{1}{1000} \times \frac{60}{1} = \frac{1}{50} \times \frac{3}{1} = \frac{3}{50}$$

$$\frac{^1/_{100}x}{^1/_{100}} = \frac{^3/_{50}}{^1/_{100}} = \frac{3}{50} \div \frac{1}{100} = \frac{3}{50} \times \frac{100}{1} = 6$$

   $x = 6$

PROOF: $^1/_{1000} \times 60 = ^3/_{50}$
$^1/_{100} \times 6 = ^3/_{50}$

4. $^1/_4 : 500 :: x : 1000$

   $500x = ^1/_4 \times 1000$

$$500x = \frac{1}{4} \times \frac{1000}{1} = 250$$

$$\frac{500x}{500} = \frac{250}{500} = 250 \div 500 = 0.5$$

   $x = 0.5$

PROOF: $500 \times 0.5 = 250$
$^1/_4 \times 1000 = 250$

5. $36 : 12 :: ^1/_{100} : x$

   $36x = 12 \times ^1/_{100}$

$$36x = \frac{12}{1} \times \frac{1}{100} = \frac{3}{25}$$

$$\frac{36x}{36} = \frac{^3/_{25}}{36} = \frac{3}{25} \div 36 = \frac{3}{25} \times \frac{1}{36} = \frac{1}{300}$$

   $x = ^1/_{300}$

PROOF: $36 \times ^1/_{300} = ^3/_{25}$
$12 \times ^1/_{100} = ^3/_{25}$

6. $6 : 24 :: 0.75 : x$

   $6x = 24 \times 0.75 = 18$

   $6x = 18$

$$\frac{6x}{6} = \frac{18}{6} = 18 \div 6 = 3$$

   $x = 3$

PROOF: $24 \times 0.75 = 18$
$6 \times 3 = 18$

7. $x : 600 :: 4 : 120$

   $120x = 4 \times 600 = 2400$

$$\frac{120x}{120} = \frac{2400}{120} = 2400 \div 120 = 20$$

   $x = 20$

PROOF: $600 \times 4 = 2400$
$20 \times 120 = 2400$

8. $0.7 : 70 :: x : 1000$

$70x = 0.7 \times 1000 = 700$

$$\frac{\cancel{70}x}{\cancel{70}} = \frac{700}{70} = 700 \div 70 = 10$$

$x = 10$

PROOF: $70 \times 10 = 700$

$0.7 \times 1000 = 700$

9. $9 : 27 :: 300 : x$

$9x = 27 \times 300 = 8100$

$$\frac{\cancel{9}x}{\cancel{9}} = \frac{8100}{9} = 8100 \div 9 = 900$$

$x = 900$

PROOF: $27 \times 300 = 8100$

$9 \times 900 = 8100$

10. $6 : 12 :: \frac{1}{4} : x$

$6x = 12 \times \frac{1}{4} = 3$

$$\frac{\cancel{6}x}{\cancel{6}} = \frac{3}{6} = 3 \div 6 = 0.5$$

$x = 0.5$

PROOF: $12 \times \frac{1}{4} = 3$

$6 \times 0.5 = 3$

☐ 2C (p. 32)

1. $\frac{1}{200} : x :: 1 : 800$

$1x = \frac{1}{200} \times 800$

$$1x = \frac{1}{200} \times \frac{800}{1} = 4$$

$$\frac{\cancel{1}x}{\cancel{1}} = \frac{4}{1} = 4 \div 1 = 4$$

$x = 4$

PROOF: $4 \times 1 = 4$

$\frac{1}{200} \times 800 = 4$

2. $15 : 30 :: x : 12$

$30x = 15 \times 12$

$30x = 180$

$$\frac{\cancel{30}x}{\cancel{30}} = \frac{180}{30} = 180 \div 30 = 6$$

$x = 6$

PROOF: $30 \times 6 = 180$

$15 \times 12 = 180$

3. $\frac{1}{1000} : \frac{1}{100} :: x : 30$

   $\frac{1}{100}x = \frac{1}{1000} \times 30$

   $$\frac{1}{100x} = \frac{1}{1000} \times \frac{30}{1} = \frac{3}{100}$$

   $$\frac{\frac{1}{100}x}{\frac{1}{100}} = \frac{\frac{3}{100}}{\frac{1}{100}} = \frac{3}{100} \div \frac{1}{100} = \frac{3}{100} \times \frac{100}{1} = 3$$

   $x = 3$

4. $6 : 12 :: 0.25 : x$

   $6x = 12 \times 0.25 = 3$

   $$\frac{6x}{6} = \frac{3}{6} = 3 \div 6 = 0.5$$

   $x = 0.5$

5. $300 : 5 :: x : \frac{1}{60}$

   $5x = \frac{1}{60} \times 300$

   $$5x = \frac{1}{60} \times \frac{300}{1} = 5$$

   $$\frac{5x}{5} = \frac{5}{5} = 5 \div 5 = 1$$

   $x = 1$

6. $\frac{1}{150} : \frac{1}{200} :: 2 : x$

   $\frac{1}{150}x = \frac{1}{200} \times 2$

   $$\frac{1}{150x} = \frac{1}{200} \times \frac{2}{1} = \frac{1}{100}$$

   $$\frac{\frac{1}{150}x}{\frac{1}{150}} = \frac{\frac{1}{100}}{\frac{1}{150}} = \frac{1}{100} \div \frac{1}{150} = \frac{1}{100} \times \frac{150}{1} = \frac{3}{2} = 1\frac{1}{2}$$

   $x = 1\frac{1}{2}$

7. $\frac{1}{2} : \frac{1}{6} :: \frac{1}{4} : x$

   $\frac{1}{2}x = \frac{1}{6} \times \frac{1}{4} = \frac{1}{24}$

   $$\frac{\frac{1}{2}x}{\frac{1}{2}} = \frac{\frac{1}{24}}{\frac{1}{2}} = \frac{1}{24} \div \frac{1}{2} = \frac{1}{24} \times \frac{2}{1} = \frac{1}{12}$$

   $x = \frac{1}{12}$

8. $7.5:12::x:28$

$12x = 7.5 \times 28 = 210$

$\dfrac{\cancel{12}x}{\cancel{12}} = \dfrac{210}{12} = 210 \div 12 = 17.5$

$x = 17.5$

9. $15:x::1.5:10$

$1.5x = 15 \times 10 = 150$

$\dfrac{\cancel{1.5}x}{\cancel{1.5}} = \dfrac{150}{1.5} = 150 \div 1.5 = 100$

$x = 100$

10. $10:x::0.4:12$

$0.4x = 10 \times 12 = 120$

$\dfrac{\cancel{.4}x}{\cancel{.4}} = \dfrac{120}{.4} = 120 \div .4 = 300$

$x = 300$

□ **2D**   (p. 33)

1. **Have**   **Want to know**

Scoops:Cups::Scoops:Cups

$4:6::x:18$

$6x = 72$

$\dfrac{\cancel{6}x}{\cancel{6}} = \dfrac{72}{6} = 12$

$x = 12$ scoops of cocoa

REMEMBER: Scoops:Cups::Scoops:Cups

Apples:Bananas::Apples:Bananas

Miles:Gallons::Miles:Gallons

You want x to stand alone. To get x to stand alone, divide by 6. Whatever you do on one side of an equation, you must do on the other.

Obtain proof by putting your answer back into the equation in place of x. Multiply the two inside numbers, and they should equal the two outside numbers.

2. **Have**   **Want to know**

Scoops:Cups::Scoops:Cups

$7:8::x:40$

$8x = 40 \times 7 = 280$

$$\frac{\cancel{8}x}{\cancel{8}} = \frac{280}{8} = 35$$

$x = 35$ scoops

PROOF: $7:8::35:40$

$8 \times 35 = 280$

$7 \times 40 = 280$

3. **Have**   **Want to know**

Bananas:Apples::Bananas:Apples

$6:9::x:72$

$9x = 6 \times 72 = 432$

$$\frac{\cancel{9}x}{\cancel{9}} = \frac{432}{9} = 48$$

$x = 48$ bananas

PROOF: $6:9::48:72$

$9 \times 48 = 432$

$6 \times 72 = 432$

4. **Have**   **Want to know**

300 mg:1 tab.::450 mg:x tab.

$300x = 450$

$$\frac{\cancel{300}x}{\cancel{300}} = \frac{450}{300} = 1.5$$

$x = 1.5$ tab.

Always label your answer.

PROOF: $300:1::450:1.5$

$1 \times 450 = 450$

$300 \times 1.5 = 450$

5. **Have**   **Want to know**

Bushes:Trees::Bushes:Trees

$8:2::x:36$

$2x = 8 \times 36 = 288$

$$\frac{\cancel{2}x}{\cancel{2}} = \frac{288}{2} = 144$$

$x = 144$ bushes

PROOF: $8:2::144:36$

$8 \times 36 = 288$

$2 \times 144 = 288$

6. **Have**   **Want to know**

Cups:Day::Cups:Day

$4:1::84:x$

$4x = 84$

$$\frac{\cancel{4}x}{\cancel{4}} = \frac{84}{4} = 21$$

$x = 21$ days

PROOF: $4:1::84:21$

$1 \times 84 = 84$

$4 \times 21 = 84$

7. **Have**   **Want to know**

Cups:Loaves::Cups:Loaves

$4:3::24:x$

$4x = 72$

$$\frac{\cancel{4}x}{\cancel{4}} = \frac{72}{4} = 18$$

$x = 18$ loaves

PROOF: $4:3::24:18$

$4 \times 18 = 72$

$3 \times 24 = 72$

8. 3 soda:$\frac{1}{2}$ fruit juice::x soda:2 fruit juice

$\frac{1}{2}x = 3 \times 2$

$$\frac{\frac{1}{2}x}{\frac{1}{2}} = \frac{6}{\frac{1}{2}} = 12$$

$x = 12$ cups soda

PROOF: $3:\frac{1}{2}::12:2$

$3 \times 2 = 6$

$\frac{1}{2} \times 12 = 6$

9. 4 tbsp sugar:1 glass::x tbsp sugar:6 glasses

$x = 6 \times 4 = 24$

$x = 24$ tbsp sugar

PROOF: $4:1::24:6$

$4 \times 6 = 24$

$1 \times 24 = 24$

10. 4 capsules:1 day::x capsules:14 days

$x = 4 \times 14 = 56$

$x = 56$ capsules

PROOF: $4:1::56:14$

$4 \times 14 = 56$

$1 \times 56 = 56$

☐ **2E**   (p. 35)

1. **Have**   **Need**

5 mg:1 tab.::40 mg:x tab.

$5x = 40$

$x = 8$ tab.

PROOF: $40 \times 1 = 40$

$5 \times 8 = 40$

2. a. More: $\frac{1}{4}$ is more than $\frac{1}{6}$.

   b. $\frac{1}{6}$ gr:1 tab.::$\frac{1}{4}$ gr:x tab.

   $\frac{1}{6}x = \frac{1}{4}$

   To get x to stand alone, divide the number by itself:

   $$\frac{\frac{1}{6}x}{\frac{1}{6}} = \frac{\cancel{\frac{1}{6}}x}{\cancel{\frac{1}{6}}} = x$$

What you do to one side you must do to the other side of the equation. Now put ⅙ under ¼. This means:

$$x = \frac{¼}{⅙} \text{ or } \frac{1}{4} \div \frac{1}{6}$$

PROOF: ⅙ × 1½ = ¼

    1 × ¼ = ¼

The problem now looks like this:

$$\frac{\cancel{⅙}x}{\cancel{⅙}} = \frac{¼}{⅙} = \frac{1}{4} \div \frac{1}{6} = \frac{1}{4} \times \frac{6}{1} = \frac{3}{2} = 1½$$

$$x = 1½ \text{ tab.}$$

3. ⅛ gr:1 tab.::⅙ gr:x tab.

   a. More: ⅙ is more than ⅛.

   b. ⅛x = ⅙

PROOF: ⅛ × 1⅓ = ⅙

     1 × ⅙ = ⅙

$$\frac{\cancel{⅛}x}{\cancel{⅛}} = \frac{⅙}{⅛} = \frac{1}{6} \div \frac{1}{8} = \frac{1}{6} \times \frac{8}{1} = 1⅓$$

$$x = 1⅓ \text{ tab.}$$

4. 3 water:2 apples::24 water:x apples

   3x = 48

PROOF: 3:2::24:16

     3 × 16 = 48

     2 × 24 = 48

$$\frac{\cancel{3}x}{\cancel{3}} = \frac{48}{3} = 16$$

$$x = 16 \text{ apples}$$

5. 6 pens:8 pencils::x pens:72 pencils

   8x = 432

PROOF: 6:8::54:72

     6 × 72 = 432

     8 × 54 = 432

$$\frac{\cancel{8}x}{\cancel{8}} = \frac{432}{8} = 54$$

$$x = 54 \text{ pens}$$

6. ½ tsp salt:3 eggs::x tsp salt:30 eggs

   3x = 30 × ½

PROOF: ½:3::5:30

     3 × 5 = 15

     ½ × 30 = 15

$$3x = \frac{30}{1} \times \frac{1}{2} = \frac{30}{2} = 15$$

$$\frac{\cancel{3}x}{\cancel{3}} = \frac{15}{3} = 5$$

$$x = 5 \text{ tsp salt}$$

7. 8 cups:7 scoops::24 cups:x scoops

    $8x = 7 \times 24$

    $\dfrac{\cancel{8}x}{\cancel{8}} = \dfrac{168}{8} = 21$

    $x = 21$ scoops

PROOF: 8:7::24:21

    $8 \times 21 = 168$

    $7 \times 24 = 168$

8. **Have**   **Want to know**

    Carnations:Ferns::Carnations:Ferns

    $5:1::x:10$

    $x = 5 \times 10$

    $x = 50$ carnations

PROOF: 5:1::50:10

    $5 \times 10 = 50$

    $1 \times 50 = 50$

9. **Have**   **Want to know**

    Vinegar:Water::Vinegar:Water

    $2:1::x:10$

    $x = 2 \times 10$

    $x = 20$ tbsp vinegar

PROOF: 2:1::20:10

    $2 \times 10 = 20$

    $1 \times 20 = 20$

10. **Have**   **Want to know**

    mg:capsule::mg:capsule

    $250:1::500:x$

    $250x = 500$

    $\dfrac{\cancel{250}x}{\cancel{250}} = \dfrac{500}{250}$

    $x = 2$ capsules

PROOF: 250:1::500:2

    $250 \times 2 = 500$

    $1 \times 500 = 500$

CHAPTER 2

Ratio and Proportion Test   (p. 37)

1. 540
2. 3
3. 12
4. 20

5. 9000
6. 10
7. 900

8. 0.5 or ½
9. 1000
10. 8⅓

Metric system

☐ **3A**   (p. 40)

1. 1000 mg	8. 100 mg	15. 15 g
2. 2000 mg	9. 1100 mg	16. 0.010 g
3. 1500 mg	10. 300 mg	17. 0.100 g
4. 500 mg	11. 0.025 g	18. 0.0005 g
5. 500 mg	12. 0.005 g	19. 0.0075 g
6. 250 mg	13. 3 g	20. 0.02015 g
7. 50 mg	14. 1.5 g	

☐ **3B**   (p. 41)

1. **Know   Want to know**

   1000 mg:1 g::25 mg:x g

   $$\frac{\cancel{1000}x}{\cancel{1000}} = \frac{25}{1000} = 25 \div 1000$$

   $x = 0.025$ g

   PROOF: $1000 \times 0.025 = 25$
   $1 \times 25 = 25$

2. **Know   Want to know**

   1000 mg:1 g::x mg:0.064 g
   $1x = 1000 \times 0.064$
   $x = 64$ mg

   PROOF: $1 \times 64 = 64$
   $1000 \times 0.064 = 64$

3. **Know   Want to know**

   1000 mg:1 g::4 mg:x g
   $1000x = 4$

   $$\frac{\cancel{1000}x}{\cancel{1000}} = \frac{4}{1000} = 4 \div 1000$$

   $x = 0.004$ g

   PROOF: $1000 \times 0.004 = 4$
   $1 \times 4 = 4$

4. **Know   Want to know**

   1000 mg:1 g::x mg:4.6 g
   $1x = 1000 \times 4.6$
   $x = 4600$ mg

   PROOF: $1 \times 4600 = 4600$
   $1000 \times 4.6 = 4600$

5. **Know**   **Want to know**

     1000 ml:1 L::375 ml:x L

     $1000x = 375$

$$\frac{\cancel{1000}x}{\cancel{1000}} = \frac{375}{1000} = 375 \div 1000$$

     $x = 0.375$ L

                                       PROOF: $0.375 \times 1000 = 375$
                                                  $1 \times 375 = 375$

6. **Know**   **Want to know**

     1000 g:1 kg::x g:89 kg

     $1x = 89{,}000$

     $x = 89{,}000$ g

                                         PROOF: $1 \times 89{,}000 = 89{,}000$
                                                  $1000 \times 89 = 89{,}000$

7. **Know**   **Want to know**

     1000 mg:1 g::45 mg:x g

     $1000x = 45$

$$\frac{\cancel{1000}x}{\cancel{1000}} = \frac{45}{1000} = 45 \div 1000$$

     $x = 0.045$ g

                                         PROOF: $1000 \times 0.045 = 45$
                                                  $1 \times 45 = 45$

8. **Know**   **Want to know**

     1000 mg:1 g::x mg:0.6 g

     $1x = 1000 \times 0.6$

     $x = 600$ mg

                                         PROOF: $1 \times 600 = 600$
                                                   $1000 \times 0.6 = 600$

9. **Know**   **Want to know**

     1 kg:2.2 lb::50 kg:x lb

     $1x = 50 \times 2.2$

     $x = 110$ lb

                                         PROOF: $2.2 \times 50 = 110$
                                                   $1 \times 110 = 110$

10. **Know**   **Want to know**

     1000 g:2.2 lb::2500 g:x lb

     $1000x = 2.2 \times 2500 = 5500$

     $x = 5.5$ lb

                                         PROOF: $2.2 \times 2500 = 5500$
                                                   $1000 \times 5.5 = 5500$

1. *Step 1:*

   Know   **Want to know**

   1000 mg:1 g::x mg:0.75 g

   $1x = 750$

   $x = 750$ mg

   PROOF: $1000 \times 0.75 = 750$

   $1 \times 750 = 750$

   Must change g into mg because that is what is available.

   Step 2:

   Know or have   Want to know

   250 mg:1 tab.::750 mg:x tab.

   $\dfrac{\cancel{250}x}{\cancel{250}} = \dfrac{750}{250} = 750 \div 250$

   $x = 3$ tab.

   PROOF: $250 \times 3 = 750$

   $1 \times 750 = 750$

   You must give 3 tablets of 250 mg each to give required amount of 750 mg.

2. *Step 1:*

   Know   **Want to know**

   1000 mg:1 g::10 mg:x g

   $1000x = 10$

   $x = 0.01$ g

   PROOF: $1000 \times 0.01 = 10$

   $1 \times 10 = 10$

   Step 2:

   Know or have   Want to know

   0.005 g:1 tab.::0.01 g:x tab.

   $\dfrac{\cancel{0.005}x}{\cancel{0.005}} = \dfrac{0.01}{0.005}$

   $x = 2$ tab. of 0.005 g

   PROOF: $1 \times 0.01 = 0.01$

   $0.005 \times 2 = 0.01$

3. *Step 1:*

   Know   **Want to know**

   1000 mg:1 g::3 mg:x g

   $1000x = 3$

   $x = 0.003$ g

   PROOF: $1 \times 3 = 3$

   $1000 \times 0.003 = 3$

Step 2:

Know or have   Want to know

0.002 g:1 tab.::0.003 g:x tab.

$0.002x = 0.003$

$x = 1.5$ tab.

PROOF: $1 \times 0.003 = 0.003$

$\qquad 0.002 \times 1.5 = 0.003$

You will give 1½ tablets of 0.002g

4. *Step 1:*

Know   Want to know

1000 mg:1 g::75 mg:x g

$1000x = 75$

$x = 0.075$ g

PROOF: $1 \times 75 = 75$

$\qquad 1000 \times 0.075 = 75$

Step 2:

Know or have   Want to know

0.050 g:1 ml::0.075 g:x ml

$0.050x = 0.075$

$x = 1.5$ ml or 1½ ml

PROOF: $1 \times 0.075 = 0.075$

$\qquad 0.050 \times 1.5 = 0.075$

5. *Step 1:*

Know   Want to know

1000 mg:1 g::x mg:0.075 g

$1x = 75$ mg

$x = 75$ mg

PROOF: $1 \times 75 = 75$

$\qquad 1000 \times 0.075 = 75$

Step 2:

Know or have   Want to know

25 mg:1 ml::75 mg:x ml

$25x = 75$

$x = 3$ ml

PROOF: $1 \times 75 = 75$

$\qquad 25 \times 3 = 75$

6. *Step 1:*

Know   Want to know

1000 mg:1 g::x mg:2 g

$1x = 2000$

$x = 2000$ mg

PROOF: $1 \times 2000 = 2000$

$\qquad 1000 \times 2 = 2000$

Step 2:

Know or have Want to know

500 mg:1 ml::2000 mg:x ml   PROOF: $1 \times 2000 = 2000$
$500x = 2000$ $500 \times 4 = 2000$
$x = 4$ ml

7. *Step 1:*

Know   Want to know

1000 mg:1 g::500 mg:x g   PROOF: $1 \times 500 = 500$
$1000x = 500$ $1000 \times 0.5 = 500$
$x = 0.5$ g

Step 2:

Know or have Want to know

0.25 g:1 tab.::0.5 g:x tab.   PROOF: $1 \times 0.5 = 0.5$
$0.25x = 0.5$ $0.25 \times 2 = 0.5$
$x = 2$ tab.

8. *Step 1:*

Know   Want to know

1000 mg:1 g::x mg:0.125 g   PROOF: $1000 \times 0.125 = 125$
$1x = 125$ $1 \times 125 = 125$
$x = 125$ mg

Step 2:

Know or have Want to know

50 mg:5 ml::125 mg:x ml   PROOF: $50 \times 12.5 = 625$
$50x = 625$ $5 \times 125 = 625$
$x = 12.5$ ml of Keflin IV

9. *Step 1:*

Know   Want to know

1000 mg:1 g::x mg:.002 g   PROOF: $1000 \times .002 = 2$
$x = 2$ mg $2 \times 1 = 2$

Step 2:

Know or have Want to know

1 mg:1 tab.::2 mg:x tab.   PROOF: $1 \times 2 = 2$
$x = 2$ tab. $2 \times 1 = 2$

10. **Know or have Want to know**

5 mg : 2 ml :: 2 mg : x ml
$5x = 4$
$x = 0.8$ ml

PROOF: $2 \times 2 = 4$
$5 \times 0.8 = 4$

CHAPTER 3

Metric System Test   (p. 45)

---

1. 0.5 g
2. 0.025 g
3. 0.005 g
4. 200 mg
5. 4000 mg

6. ½ tab. (two-step problem)
7. 3 tab. (one-step problem)
8. 3 tab. (two-step problem)
9. 2 tab.
10. 2 tab.

CHAPTER 4

Apothecary system

☐ **4A**   (p. 50)

REMEMBER: *Have* or *know* goes on the left.

1. **Have   Want to know**

gr ½ : 1 ml :: gr 1 : x ml

$$\frac{\frac{1}{2}x}{\frac{1}{2}} = \frac{1}{\frac{1}{2}} = 1 \div \frac{1}{2} = 1 \times 2 = 2$$

$x = 2$ ml

PROOF: $\frac{1}{2} \times 2 = 1$
$1 \times 1 = 1$

2. **Have   Want to know**

gr 5 : 1 tab. :: gr 15 : x tab.
$5x = 15$
$x = 3$ tab.

PROOF: $5 \times 3 = 15$
$1 \times 15 = 15$

3. **Have   Want to know**

gr ⅛ : 1 ml :: gr ⅙ : x ml

$$\frac{\frac{1}{8}x}{\frac{1}{8}} = \frac{\frac{1}{6}}{\frac{1}{8}} = \frac{1}{6} \div \frac{1}{8} = \frac{1}{6} \times \frac{8}{1} = \frac{4}{3} = 1\frac{1}{3}$$

$x = 1\frac{1}{3}$ ml

PROOF: $\frac{1}{8} \times 1\frac{1}{3} = \frac{1}{6}$
$1 \times \frac{1}{6} = \frac{1}{6}$

$$\text{Answer must be a decimal. Therefore: } 1\frac{1}{3} = \frac{4}{3} = 3\overline{)4.00} \quad \begin{array}{r} 1.33 = 1.33 \\ \hline \end{array}$$

$$\begin{array}{r} \underline{3} \\ 1\,0 \\ \underline{9} \\ 10 \\ \underline{9} \\ 1 \end{array}$$

Give 1.3 ml of morphine sulfate.

4. **Have**   **Want to know**

gr 7.5:1 suppository::gr 15:x suppositories

PROOF: $7.5 \times 2 = 15$
$1 \times 15 = 15$

$$\frac{7.5x}{7.5} = \frac{15}{7.5} = 15 \div 7.5 = \frac{15}{1} \times \frac{1}{7.5} = \frac{15}{7.5} = 2$$

$x = 2$ suppositories
Give 2 suppositories.

5. This is a two-step problem. You must find out what part ʒ i (dr) is to ℥ i (oz).

Know   **Want to know**

ʒ ī:1 tsp::ʒ īī:x tsp

PROOF: $1 \times 2 = 2$
$1 \times 2 = 2$

$x = 1 \times 2 = 2$
$x = 2$ tsp

Know   **Want to know**

1 tsp:5 ml::2 tsp:x ml

PROOF: $1 \times 10 = 10$
$5 \times 2 = 10$

$x = 5 \times 2 = 10$
$x = 10$ ml

6. What do you know about ℥ and ml?

Know   **Want to know**

30 ml:1 oz::x ml:½ oz

PROOF: $30 \times \frac{1}{2} = 15$
$1 \times 15 = 15$

$$1x = 30 \times \frac{1}{2} = 15$$

$x = 15$ ml of Maalox

The fact that the bottle contained 8 oz of Maalox has nothing to do with the relationship between ml and 1 oz.

7. Give less than 1 ml.

Have   **Want to know**

gr ¼:1 ml::gr ⅙: x ml

$$\frac{1}{4}x = \frac{1}{6}$$

$$\frac{1}{6} \div \frac{1}{4} = \frac{1}{6} \times \frac{4}{1} = \frac{2}{3}$$

$x = \frac{2}{3}$ ml

PROOF: ¼ × ⅔ = ⅙

          1 × ⅙ = ⅙

Answer must be a decimal.
$$\frac{2}{3} = 3\overline{)2.00} \quad .66$$
$$\underline{1\ 8}$$
$$20$$
$$\underline{18}$$
$$2$$

Give 0.66 ml of codeine sulfate SC.

8. **Have**   **Want to know**

gr ½:1 capsule::gr 1½: x capsules

½x = 1½

$$\frac{½x}{½} = \frac{3/2}{½}$$

3/2 × 2/1 = 6/2 = 3

Give 3 capsules

PROOF: ½ × 3 = 1½

          1 × 1½ = 1½

9. **Have**   **Want to have**

gr 2:1.25 ml::gr 3: x ml

2x = 3 × 1.25 or 3.75

$$\frac{2x}{2} = \frac{3.75}{2} = 1.875$$

x = 1.9 ml

Give 1.9 ml

PROOF: 2 × 1.9 = 3.8

          1.25 × 3 = 3.75 or 3.8

10. **Have**   **Want to have**

gr 1½:1 capsule::gr 3: x caps

1½x = 3

$$\frac{1½x}{1½} = \frac{3}{1½} \text{ or } 3 \times \frac{2}{3} = 2$$

x = 2 capsules

Give 2 capsules

PROOF: 1½ × 2 = 3

          1 × 3 = 3

1. This is a two-step problem. First find out how many ml you are to give. Then figure how many minims per ml.

   Have   **Want to know**

   gr $\frac{1}{10}$:1 ml::gr $\frac{1}{8}$:x ml

   $$\frac{\cancel{\frac{1}{10}}x}{\cancel{\frac{1}{10}}} = \frac{\frac{1}{8}}{\frac{1}{10}} = \frac{1}{8} \div \frac{1}{10} = \frac{1}{8} \times \frac{10}{1} = \frac{5}{4} = 1\frac{1}{4}$$

   $x = 1\frac{1}{4}$ ml

   PROOF: $1\frac{1}{4} \times \frac{1}{10} = \frac{1}{8}$

   $1 \times \frac{1}{8} = \frac{1}{8}$

   Because your problem is not completed, you may leave answer in fraction form or change it to a decimal.

   You must memorize that there are 15 to 16 minims in 1 ml.

   Have   **Want to know**

   16 ℳ:1 ml::xℳ:1$\frac{1}{4}$ ml

   $$1x = \frac{16}{1} \times \frac{5}{4} = \frac{80}{4} = 20$$

   $x = 20$ minims

   PROOF: $16 \times 1\frac{1}{4} = 20$

   $1 \times 20 = 20$

2. **Know**   **Want to know**

   8 ℥ (dr):1℥ (oz)::x ℥:$\frac{1}{4}$ ℥

   $$1x = \frac{8}{1} \times \frac{1}{4} = \frac{8}{4} = 2$$

   $x = 2$ dr

   PROOF: $8 \times \frac{1}{4} = 2$

   $1 \times 2 = 2$

3. This is a two-step problem.

   Have   **Want to know**

   gr $\frac{1}{150}$:$\frac{1}{2}$ ml::gr $\frac{1}{200}$:x ml

   $$\frac{1}{150}x = \frac{1}{2} \times \frac{1}{200} = \frac{1}{400}$$

   $$\frac{\cancel{\frac{1}{150}}x}{\cancel{\frac{1}{150}}} = \frac{\frac{1}{400}}{\frac{1}{150}} = \frac{1}{400} \times \frac{150}{1} = \frac{3}{8}$$

   $x = 0.37$ ml

   PROOF: $\frac{1}{2} \times \frac{1}{200} = \frac{1}{400}$

   $\frac{1}{150} \times \frac{3}{8} = \frac{1}{400}$

   You may either change fraction to decimal or leave it as it is for working out the remainder of the problem.

Know	Want to know	

16 ℳ:1 ml::x ℳ:⅜ ml

$$1x = \frac{16}{1} \times \frac{3}{8} = \frac{48}{8} = 6$$

$x = 6$ minims

PROOF: $1 \times 6 = 6$

$16 \times ⅜ = 6$

4. **Have**   **Want to know**

gr 5:1 tab.::gr 15:x tab.
$5x = 15$
$x = 3$ tab.

PROOF: $5 \times 3 = 15$

$1 \times 15 = 15$

5. **Know**   **Want to know**

℥ i̅:8 ℥::℥ s̅s̅:x ℥

$$x = 8 \times \frac{1}{2} = \frac{8}{2} = 4$$

$x = 4$ dr

PROOF: $1 \times 4 = 4$

$8 \times ½ = 4$

Know   **Want to know**

℥ i̅:5 ml::℥ i̅v:x ml
$x = 5 \times 4 = 20$
$x = 20$ ml

PROOF: $1 \times 20 = 20$

$5 \times 4 = 20$

CHAPTER 4

Apothecary System Test (p. 53)

1. 0.5 ml
2. 0.75 ml
3. 0.66 ml
4. 15 ml
5. 0.5 ml
6. 0.37 ml and 4.44 ℳ
7. 0.5 ml
8. 3 tab.
9. 2 capsules
10. 2 capsules

Apothecary and metric conversions

□ **5A**   (p. 57)

1. **Know**   **Want to know**

   1.0 g:gr 15::x g:gr 10   PROOF: $15 \times 0.66 = 9.9 = 10$
   $15x = 10 = 10 \div 15 = 0.66$ $1 \times 10 = 10$
   $x = 0.66$g

2. **Know**   **Want to know**

   1.0 g:gr 15::0.5 g:gr x PROOF: $15 \times 0.5 = 7.5$
   $1x = 15 \times 0.5 = 7.5$ $1 \times 7.5 = 7.5$
   $x = $ gr 7.5

3. **Know**   **Want to know**

   1.0 g:gr 15::x g:gr 30   PROOF: $15 \times 2 = 30$
   $15x = 30$ $1 \times 30 = 30$
   $x = 2$ g

4. **Know**   **Want to know**

   1.0 g:gr 15::0.1 g:gr x PROOF: $15 \times 0.1 = 1.5$
   $1x = 1.5$ $1 \times 1.5 = 1.5$
   $x = $ gr 1.5

5. **Know**   **Want to know**

   1.0 g:gr 15::x g:gr 7½   PROOF: $15 \times 0.5 = 7.5$
   $15x = 7½$ $1 \times 7.5 = 7.5$
   $x = 0.5$ g

6. **Know**   **Want to know**

   1.0 g:gr 15::3.0 g:gr x PROOF: $15 \times 3.0 = 45$
   $1.0x = 45.0$ $1.0 \times 45.0 = 45$
   $x = $ gr 45.0

7. **Know**   **Want to know**

   60.0 mg:gr i::x mg:gr ¾   PROOF: $1 \times 45 = 45$
   $1x = 60 \times ¾ = 45$ $60 \times ¾ = 45$
   $x = 45$ mg

8. **Know** **Want to know**

60 mg:gr i::60 mg:gr x

$60x = 60$

$x = $ gr 1

PROOF: $1 \times 60 = 60$

$60 \times 1 = 60$

9. **Know** **Want to know**

60 mg:gr 1::x mg:gr ¼

$1x = 60 \times ¼ = 15$

$x = 15$ mg

PROOF: $1 \times 15 = 15$

$60 \times ¼ = 15$

10. **Know** **Want to know**

60 mg:gr 1::x mg:gr ¹⁄₁₅₀

$1x = 60 \times \dfrac{1}{150} = ⅖ = 5\overline{)2.0}$

$\phantom{1x = 60 \times \dfrac{1}{150} = ⅖ = 5)}\underline{2\ 0}$

$x = 0.4$ mg

PROOF: $1 \times 0.4 = 0.4$

$60 \times ¹⁄₁₅₀ = ⅖ = 0.4$

□ **5B** (p. 58)

Use conversion tables for proof.

1. 0.001 g
2. 5000 mg
3. gr 15
4. 0.5 g
5. gr ¼
6. 1000 ml
7. 1 oz

8. 15 to 16 gtt
9. 8 ml
10. 1 ml
11. 1000 g
12. 0.3 mg
13. 180 mg
14. 30 ml

15. 5 ml
16. 1 ℳ
17. Milligrams are smaller than grains (gr i = 60 mg)
18. g
19. 30 ml
20. 15 ml

□ **5C** (p. 58)

REMEMBER: *Know* and *have* go on the *left*.

1. ℥ i:30 ml::℥ 1½:x ml

$1x = 30 \times 1½ = \dfrac{30}{1} \times \dfrac{3}{2} = 45$

$x = 45$ ml

PROOF: $30 \times 1½ = 45$

$1 \times 45 = 45$

2. This is a two-step problem. Must change gr $\frac{1}{300}$ to mg because that is what you have on hand.

Know   **Want to know**

60 mg:gr i:: x mg:gr $\frac{1}{300}$

$$1x = \frac{1}{300} \times \frac{60}{1} = \frac{1}{5}$$

$x = \frac{1}{5}$ mg   Change $\frac{1}{5}$ to a decimal because mg is a metric measure and metric is a decimal system; so:
$1 \div 5 = 0.2$ mg.

PROOF: $1 \times \frac{1}{5} = \frac{1}{5}$
$60 \times \frac{1}{300} = \frac{1}{5}$

Have   **Want to know**

0.5 mg:0.5 ml::0.2 mg:x ml

$0.50x = 0.10$

$x = 0.2$ ml   Give 0.2 ml of atropine.

PROOF: $0.50 \times 0.2 = 0.1$
$0.5 \times 0.2 = 0.1$

NOTE: Do *not* round off ml or cc to whole numbers. Syringes are marked to give tenths and hundredths. Check the calibrations on your syringes.

3. **Know**   **Want to know**

5 ml:1 ℨ::x ml:2 ℨ

$x = 10$ ml

PROOF: $5 \times 2 = 10$
$1 \times 10 = 10$

4. **Know**   **Want to know**

60 mg:gr i::x mg:gr $\frac{3}{4}$

$1x = 60 \times \frac{3}{4} = 45$

$x = 45$ mg

PROOF: $1 \times 45 = 45$
$60 \times \frac{3}{4} = 45$

Have   **Want to know**

75 mg:1 ml::45 mg:x ml

$75x = 45$

$x = 0.6$ ml

PROOF: $1 \times 45 = 45$
$75 \times 0.6 = 45$

5. **Know**   **Want to know**

1 gr:gr 15::0.6 g:gr x

$1x = 9$

$x = $ gr 9

PROOF: $15 \times 0.6 = 9$
$1 \times 9 = 9$

Have   **Want to know**

gr 5:1 tab.::gr 9:x tab.

$5x = 9$

$x = 1.8$ tab.   Give 2 tab. of gr v each tablet.

PROOF: $1 \times 9 = 9$
$5 \times 1.8 = 9$

Can you give $\frac{8}{10}$ of a tablet? Not very easily, so the only thing to do is to give 2 tab. of gr v.

6. **Know**   **Want to know**

   60 mg:gr i::720 mg:gr x

   $60x = 720$

   $x = 12$ gr

   PROOF: $720 \times 1 = 720$

   $60 \times 12 = 720$

   Have   **Want to know**

   gr 5:1 tab.::gr 12:x tab.

   $5x = 12$

   $x = 2.4$ tab.   Give 2½ tab. of gr 5 each.

   PROOF: $1 \times 12 = 12$

   $5 \times 2.4 = 12$

7. **Know**   **Want to know**

   1 g:gr 15::x g:gr 7½

   $15x = 7½$

   $x = 0.5$ g

   PROOF: $15 \times 0.5 = 7.5$

   $7.5 \times 1 = 7.5$

   Have   **Want to know**

   0.5 g:2.0 cc::0.5 g:x cc

   $0.5x = 1.0$

   $x = 2$ cc (ml)

   PROOF: $2 \times 0.5 = 1$

   $0.5 \times 2 = 1$

8. **Have**   **Want to know**

   gr 7½:2 ml::gr 5:x ml

   $7½x = 2 \times 5 = 10$

   $x = 1.3$ ml

   PROOF: $2 \times 5 = 10$

   $7½ \times 1⅓ = 10$

9. **Know**   **Want to know**

   60 mg:1 gr::100 mg:x gr

   $60x = 100$

   $x = 1.66$ gr

   PROOF: $60 \times 1.66 = 99.6$

   $1 \times 100 = 100$

   Have   **Want to have**

   1.5 gr:1 cap::1.6 gr:x capsules

   $1.5x = 1.6$

   $x = 1.06$ or 1 capsule

   (Remember, grains do not convert exactly to
   metric system: 60–67 mg = 1 gr.)

   PROOF: $1.5 \times 1 = 1.5$

   $1 \times 1.6 = 1.6$

10. **Know**   **Want to know**

    60 mg:1 gr::30 mg:x gr

    $60x = 30$

    $x = ½$ gr

    PROOF: $60 \times ½ = 30$

    $1 \times 30 = 30$

    2 gr:1.25 ml::½ gr:x ml

    $2x = 1.25 \times 0.5 = .625$

    (Use *either* decimals *or* fractions.
    Do not mix.)

    $x = 0.31$ ml

    PROOF: $2 \times 0.31 = 0.62$

    $1.25 \times 0.5 = 0.62$

1. **Have**   **Want to know**

   gr $\frac{1}{150}$:1 ml::gr $\frac{1}{200}$:x ml

   $\frac{1}{150}x = \frac{1}{200} = \dfrac{1}{200} \div \dfrac{1}{150} = \dfrac{1}{200} \times \dfrac{150}{1} = \frac{3}{4}$ ml

   $x = \frac{3}{4}$ ml

   Change $\frac{3}{4}$ ml to metric (decimal) 0.75.

   PROOF: $\frac{1}{150} \times \frac{3}{4} = \frac{1}{200}$

   $\ 1 \times \frac{1}{200} = \frac{1}{200}$

2. **Have**   **Want to know**

   gr $\frac{1}{4}$:1 ml::gr $\frac{1}{6}$:x ml

   $\frac{1}{4}x = \frac{1}{6}$

   $x = \frac{2}{3}$ ml or 0.66 =$_|$0.7 ml

   Change fraction to metric (decimal).

   PROOF: $1 \times \frac{1}{6} = \frac{1}{6}$

   $\ \frac{1}{4} \times \frac{2}{3} = \frac{1}{6}$

3. **Know**   **Want to know**

   60 mg:gr i::x mg:gr $\frac{1}{2}$

   $1x = 60 \times \frac{1}{2} = 30$

   $x = 30$ mg

   PROOF: $1 \times 30 = 30$

   $\ 60 \times \frac{1}{2} = 30$

   Have   **Want to know**

   15 mg:1 tab.::30 mg:x tab.

   $15x = 30$

   $x = 2$ tab.

   PROOF: $1 \times 30 = 30$

   $\ 15 \times 2 = 30$

4. **Have**   **Want to know**

   400,000 U:1 ml::300,000 U:x ml

   $\dfrac{400,000x}{400,000} = \dfrac{300,000}{400,000} = \dfrac{3}{4} = 3 \div 4 = 0.75$

   $x = 0.75$ ml

   PROOF: $1 \times 300,000 = 300,000$

   $\ 400,000 \times 0.75 = 300,000$

   Know   **Want to know**

   15 ♏:1 ml::x ♏:0.75 ml

   $1x = 15 \times 0.75 = 11.25$

   $x = 11$ minims

   PROOF: $1 \times 11 = 11$

   $\ 15 \times 0.75 = 11.25$

5. **Know**   **Want to know**

   1000 mg:1 g::x mg:0.50 g

   $1x = 500$ mg

   $x = 500$ mg

   PROOF: $1 \times 500 = 500$

   $\ 1000 \times 0.50 = 500$

Have　　　　**Want to know**

250 mg:1 tab.::500 mg:x tab.

250x = 500

x = 2 tab.

PROOF: $1 \times 500 = 500$

$250 \times 2 = 500$

6. **Have**　　　　**Want to know**

100 mg:2 ml::75 mg:x ml

100x = 150

x = 1.5 ml

PROOF: $2 \times 75 = 150$

$100 \times 1.5 = 150$

7. None. We hope you won't give scopolamine when atropine was ordered.

8. **Know**　　　**Want to know**

1 g:gr 15::x g:gr 7½

15x = 7½

$1x = \dfrac{7½}{15} = ½$

x = 0.5 g

PROOF: $15 \times 0.5 = 7.5$

$1 \times 7½ = 7½$

Have　　　　**Want to know**

0.25 g:1 tab.::0.5 g:x tab.

0.25x = 0.5

$1x = \dfrac{0.5}{0.25} = 2$

x = 2 tab.

PROOF: $1 \times 0.5 = 0.5$

$0.25 \times 2 = 0.5$

9. **Know**　　　**Want to know**

30 ml:1 oz::x ml:½ oz

$x = 30 \times ½ = {}^{30}\!/_2$

x = 15 ml

PROOF: $30 \times ½ = 15$

$1 \times 15 = 15$

10. **Know**　　　**Want to know**

60 mg:1 gr::x mg:$\frac{1}{200}$ gr

$x = \dfrac{60}{1} \times \dfrac{1}{200} = \dfrac{6\cancel{0}}{20\cancel{0}} = \dfrac{3}{10}$

x = 0.3 mg

PROOF: $60 \times \frac{1}{200} = 0.3$

$1 \times 0.3 = 0.3$

Have　　　　**Want to know**

0.4 mg:1 ml::0.3 mg:x ml

$\dfrac{\cancel{0.4}x}{\cancel{0.4}} = \dfrac{0.3}{0.4} = 0.75$

x = 0.75 ml

PROOF: $0.4 \times 0.75 = 0.3$

$1 \times 0.3 = 0.3$

☐ **5E** (p. 62)

1. **Have**   **Want to know**

   gr $\frac{1}{150}$:1 ml::gr $\frac{1}{200}$:x ml   PROOF: $1 \times \frac{1}{200} = \frac{1}{200}$

   $\frac{1}{150}x = \frac{1}{200} \div \frac{1}{150} = \frac{1}{200} \times \frac{150}{1} = \frac{3}{4}$ $\frac{1}{150} \times \frac{3}{4} = \frac{1}{200}$

   $x = \frac{3}{4} = 0.75$ ml   Give 0.75 ml of atropine.

   Know   **Want to know**

   16 ♏:1 ml::x ♏:$\frac{3}{4}$ ml   PROOF: $1 \times 12 = 12$

   $1x = 16 \times \frac{3}{4} = 12$ $16 \times \frac{3}{4} = 12$

   $x = 12$ ♏

2. **Know**   **Want to know**

   ℨ i:30 ml::ℨ $\frac{1}{2}$:x ml   PROOF: $30 \times \frac{1}{2} = 15$

   $1x = 30 \times \frac{1}{2} = 15$ $1 \times 15 = 15$

   $x = 15$ ml

   Know   **Want to know**

   15 ml:2 hours::x ml:24 hours   PROOF: $2 \times 180 = 360$

   $2x = 360$ $15 \times 24 = 360$

   $x = 180$ ml in 24 hours

3. **Know**   **Want to know**

   1 ♏:1 gtt::9 ♏:x gtt   PROOF: $9 \times 1 = 9$

   $1x = 9$ $1 \times 9 = 9$

   $x = 9$ gtt

4. **Know**   **Want to know**

   30 ml:1 oz::x ml:6 oz   PROOF: $1 \times 180 = 180$

   $1x = 180$ $6 \times 30 = 180$

   $x = 180$ ml

   Have   **Want to know**

   180 ml:6 oz::x ml:3 oz ($\frac{1}{2}$ glass)   PROOF: $6 \times 90 = 540$

   $6x = 540$ $3 \times 180 = 540$

   $x = 90$ ml

5. **Know**   **Want to know**

   4 ml:1 tsp.::8 ml:x tsp   PROOF: $1 \times 8 = 8$

   $4x = 8$ $4 \times 2 = 8$

   $x = 2$ tsp

   Know   **Want to know**

   1 dr:4 ml::x dr:8 ml   PROOF: $1 \times 8 = 8$

   $4x = 8$ $4 \times 2 = 8$

   $x = 2$ dr

6. **Have**   **Want to know**

    1 g:2 ml::0.2 g:x ml   PROOF: $1 \times 0.4 = 0.4$

    $x = 2 \times 0.2 = 0.4$ $2 \times 0.2 = 0.4$

    $x = 0.4$ ml

7. **Know**   **Want to know**

    1000 mg:1 g::x mg:0.05 g   PROOF: $1 \times 50 = 50$

    $1x = 1000 \times 0.05 = 50$ $1000 \times 0.05 = 50$

    $x = 50$ mg

    Know   **Want to know**

    100 mg:1 tab.::50 mg:x tab.   PROOF: $50 \times 1 = 50$

    $100x = 50 \div 100 = \frac{1}{2}$ $100 \times \frac{1}{2} = 50$

    $x = 0.5$ tab. or ½ tab.

8. **Know**   **Want to know**

    1000 mg:1 g::15 mg:x g   PROOF: $1000 \times 0.015 = 15$

    $1000x = 15 \div 1000 = 0.015$ $1 \times 15 = 15$

    $x = 0.015$ g

    Have   **Want to know**

    0.03 g:1 tab.::.015 g:x tab.   PROOF: $0.03 \times 0.5\ (\frac{1}{2}) = 0.015$

    $0.03x = 0.015 \div 0.03 = \frac{1}{2}$ or 0.5 $1 \times 0.015 = 0.015$

    $x = \frac{1}{2}$ tab.

9. **Know**   **Want to know**

    1000 mg:1 g::x mg: 0.05 g   PROOF: $1000 \times .05 = 50$

    $x = 1000 \times 0.05$ or 50 mg $1 \times 50 = 50$

    Have   **Want to know**

    25 mg:1 tab.::50 mg:x tab.   PROOF: $25 \times 2 = 50$

    $25x = 50$ $1 \times 50 = 50$

    $x = 2$ tab.

10. **Know**   **Want to know**

    1000 mg:1 g::x mg:0.1 g   PROOF: $1000 \times 0.1 = 100$

    $x = 1000 \times 0.1 = 100$ mg $1 \times 100 = 100$

    Have   **Want to know**

    125 mg:5 ml::100 mg:x ml   PROOF: $125 \times 4 = 500$

    $125x = 500$ $5 \times 100 = 500$

    $x = 4$ ml

Apothecary and Metric Conversions Test   (p. 64)

1. 0.67 g	5. 0.33 g	8. 9 gtt
2. gr 7½	6. 0.5 g	9. 0.66 ml
3. 2 g	7. gr 45	10. 0.25 ml
4. gr 1½		

Medications from powder and crystals

☐ **6A**   (p. 66)

1. Add 2.5 ml of sterile water for injection; 330 mg/ml.
   Refrigerated, 96 hrs; room temperature, 24 hrs.

   Have   **Want**

   330 mg:1 ml::300 mg:x ml

   $330x = 300$

   $x = 0.9$ ml

   PROOF: $330 \times 0.9 = 297$

   $\qquad\quad 300 \times 1 = 300$

2. Add 5.7 ml of sterile water for injection; 1.5 ml/250 mg.
   Refrigerated, 7 days; room temperature, 3 days.

   Have   **Want**

   250 mg:1.5 ml::450 mg:x ml

   $250x = 1.5 \times 450 = 675$

   $250x = 675$

   $x = 2.7$ ml

   PROOF: $250 \times 2.7 = 675$

   $\qquad\quad 1.5 \times 450 = 675$

3. Add 3.5 ml diluent.
   The reconstituted medication will yield 250 mg/ml.
   Use within 1 hour—very unstable medication.

   Have   **Want**

   250 mg:1 ml::500 mg:x ml

   $250x = 500$

   $x = 2$ ml

   PROOF: $1 \times 500 = 500$

   $\qquad\quad 250 \times 2 = 500$

4. Add 5.7 ml sterile water for injection.
   The reconstituted medication will yield 250 mg/1.5 ml.
   Use within 3 days at room temperature or 7 days refrigerated.

   Have   **Want**

   250 mg:1 ml::300 mg:x ml   PROOF: $1 \times 300 = 300$
   $250x = 300$ $250 \times 1.2 = 300$
   $x = 1.2$ ml

5. Add 5.7 ml of sterile water for injection.
   The reconstituted medication will yield 1 g/2 ml Staphcillin.
   Discard after 24 hours at room temperature or 4 days refrigerated.

   Have   **Want**

   1000 mg:2 ml::1000 mg:x ml   PROOF: $2 \times 1000 = 2000$
   $1000x = 2 \times 1000 = 2000$ $1000 \times 2 = 2000$
   $x = 2$ ml

6. 500,000 U/ml
   Add 1.6 ml diluent for injection.
   Refrigerated, 7 days.

   Have   **Want**

   50$\emptyset$,$\emptyset\emptyset\emptyset$ U:1.6 ml::75$\emptyset$,$\emptyset\emptyset\emptyset$ u:x ml   PROOF: $50 \times 2.4 = 120$
   $50x = 1.6 \times 75 = 120$ $1.6 \times 75 = 120$
   $50x = 120$
   $x = 2.4$

7. Add 2 ml of sterile water for injection.
   The reconstituted medication will yield 1 g/2.6 ml.
   Use medication promptly.

   Have   **Want**

   1000 mg:2.6 ml::750 mg:x ml   PROOF: $1000 \times 1.95 = 1950$
   $1000x = 2.6 \times 750 = 1950$ $2.6 \times 750 = 1950$
   $1000x = 1950$
   $x = 1.95 = 2$ ml

☐ **6B**   (p. 68)

1. **Know**   **Want**

   1 g:1000 mg::x g:500 mg   PROOF: $1000 \times 0.5 = 500$
   $1000x = 500$ $1 \times 500 = 500$
   $x = 0.5$ g

■ 173

Have   **Want**

0.25 g:1.5 ml::0.5 g:x ml

$0.25x = 1.5 \times 0.5 = 0.75$

$x = 3$ ml

PROOF: $1.5 \times 0.5 = 0.75$

$0.25 \times 3 = 0.75$

2. Make the 500,000 U per ml solution.

Have   **Want**

5̸0̸0̸,0̸0̸0̸ U:1 ml :: 3̸0̸0̸,0̸0̸0̸ U:x ml

$5x = 3$

$x = 0.6$ ml

PROOF: $1 \times 3 = 3$

$5 \times 0.6 = 3$

3. **Have**   **Want**

500 ml:2.2 ml::200 mg:x ml

$500x = 2.2 \times 200 = 440$

$x = 0.88 = 0.9$ ml

PROOF: $500 \times 0.88 = 440$

$2.2 \times 200 = 440$

4. **Have**   **Want**

1 ml:225 mg::x ml:125 mg

$225x = 125$

$x = 0.55 = 0.6$ ml

PROOF: $1 \times 125 = 125$

$225 \times 0.55 = 123.75$

5. Now that you know how to move the decimal three places to the right to change g to mg, this can be a one-step problem.

Have   **Want**

1 ml:250 mg::x ml:500 mg

$250x = 500$

$x = 2$ ml

PROOF: $1 \times 500 = 500$

$250 \times 2 = 500$

6. You know that 0.50 g = 500 mg. Therefore, dilute the entire vial of powder with 10 ml of sterile water for injection. Fill Volutrol with 90 ml of IV solution and add the 10 ml of reconstituted medication.

7. You know that 1 g = 1000 mg. Therefore, this can be a one-step problem.

Have   **Want**

1000 mg:3 ml::300 mg:x ml

$1000x = 900$

$x = 0.9$ ml

PROOF: $3 \times 300 = 900$

$1000 \times 0.9 = 900$

8. **Know**   **Want**

5̸0̸0̸,0̸0̸0̸ U:1 ml::1,2̸0̸0̸,0̸0̸0̸ U:x ml   PROOF: $1 \times 12 = 12$

$5x = 12$ $2.4 \times 5 = 12$

$x = 2.4$ ml will contain 1.2 million U of penicillin

How many ml will be left in the vial?
Vial contains 10.0 ml
Gave   <u>2.4 ml</u>
             7.6 ml remaining in vial

How many units of penicillin will be left in the vial?

Know   **Want**

500,000 U:1 ml::x U:10 ml   PROOF: $1 \times 5,000,000 = 5,000,000$

$1x = 10 \times 500,000 = 5,000,000$ $10 \times 500,000 = 5,000,000$

$x = 5$ million units in entire vial

    5,000,000 units in entire vial
<u>−1,200,000</u> units given in 2.4 ml
    3,800,000 units left in vial

9. **Have**   **Want**

5̸0̸0̸,0̸0̸0̸ U:1 ml :: 5,0̸0̸0̸,0̸0̸0̸ U:x ml   PROOF: $5 \times 10 = 50$

$5x = 50$ $1 \times 50 = 50$

$x = 10$ ml diluent needed to make 500,000 U/ml

10. **Have**   **Want**

5̸0̸0̸,0̸0̸0̸ U:1 ml::8̸0̸0̸,0̸0̸0̸ U:x ml   PROOF: $1 \times 8 = 8$

$5x = 8$ $5 \times 1.6 = 8$

$x = 1.6$ ml

CHAPTER 6

Medications From Powder and Crystals Test   (p. 71)

---

1. 0.5 ml   PROOF: $30 \times 0.5 = 15$
You may cross out zeros in equal amounts on both sides $5 \times 3 = 15$
of the equation.

2. After diluting with 4 ml of sterile water, give 2.2 ml.

3. 10 ml   PROOF: $5 \times 10 = 50$
Add 10 ml of distilled water to a vial to make 50,000 U/ml. $1 \times 50 = 50$
Label vial: date, time, and units per ml.

4. Add 4 ml distilled water to vial
   Each ml of carbenicillin will contain 250,000 U.
   Label vial: date, time, and units per ml.

   PROOF: $25 \times 4 = 100$
   $1 \times 100 = 100$

5. $0.6\frac{2}{3} = 0.7$ ml

   PROOF: $1 \times 4 = 4$
   $0.6\frac{2}{3} \times 6 = 4$

CHAPTER 7

Insulin

☐ 7A (p. 76)

1. **Know**   **Want**
   100 U:1 ml::15 U:x ml
   $100x = 15$
   $x = 0.15$ ml. Use a tuberculin syringe.

   PROOF: $1 \times 15 = 15$
   $100 \times 0.15 = 15$

2. **Know**   **Want**
   100 U:1 ml::75 U:x ml
   $100x = 75$
   $x = 0.75$ ml

   PROOF: $100 \times 0.75 = 75$
   $1 \times 75 = 75$

3. 500 U:1 ml::150 U:x ml
   $500x = 150$
   $x = 0.3$ ml

   PROOF: $500 \times 0.3 = 150$
   $1 \times 150 = 150$

4. 100 U:1 ml::45 U:x ml
   $100x = 45$
   $x = 0.45$ ml

   PROOF: $100 \times .45 = 45$
   $1 \times 45 = 45$

5. It does not state the *amount* of U 100 insulin to be given.

6. It does not state the *amount* of U 100 insulin to be given.

7. **Know**   **Want**
   100 U:1 ml::100 U:x ml
   $100x = 100$
   $x = 1$ ml

   PROOF: $100 \times 1 = 100$
   $1 \times 100 = 100$

8. On U 100 0.5 ml syringes, measure 34 units.

9. On a U 100 1 ml syringe, measure 56 units total.

10. Using a TB syringe

Have	Want
Have	**Want**

100 U:1 ml::18 U:x ml PROOF: $100 \times 0.18 = 18$
$100x = 18$ $1 \times 18 = 18$
$x = 0.18$ ml Ultralente

Have **Want**
100 U:1 ml::16 U:x ml PROOF: $100 \times 0.16 = 16$
$100x = 16$ $1 \times 16 = 16$
$x = 0.16$ ml
Give a total of 0.34 in a TB syringe.

□ 7B (p. 78)

1. **Know** **Want**
   100 U:1 ml::35 U:x ml PROOF: $100 \times 0.35 = 35$
   $100x = 35$ $1 \times 35 = 35$
   $x = 0.35$ ml

2. **Know** **Want**
   100 U:1 ml::20 U:x ml PROOF: $100 \times 0.2 = 20$
   $100x = 20$ $1 \times 20 = 20$
   $x = 0.2$ ml

3. **Know** **Want**
   100 U:1 ml::45 U:x ml PROOF: $100 \times 0.45 = 45$
   $100x = 45$ $1 \times 45 = 45$
   $x = 0.45$ ml

4. **Know** **Want**
   100 U:1 ml::65 U:x ml PROOF: $100 \times 0.65 = 65$
   $100x = 65$ $1 \times 65 = 65$
   $x = 0.65$ ml

5. **Know** **Want**
   100 U:1 ml::20 U:x ml PROOF: $100 \times 0.2 = 20$
   $100x = 20$ $1 \times 20 = 20$
   $x = 0.2$ ml

6. **Know**   **Want**

     100 U:1 ml::40 U:x ml   PROOF: $1 \times 40 = 40$

     $100x = 40$ $100 \times 0.4 = 40$

     $x = 0.4$ ml

7. **Know**   **Want**

     500 U:1 ml::160 U:x ml   PROOF: $500 \times 0.32 = 160$

     $500x = 160$ $1 \times 160 = 160$

     $x = 0.32$ ml

8. **Know**   **Want**

     100 U:1 ml::35 U:x ml   PROOF: $1 \times 35 = 35$

     $100x = 35$ $100 \times 0.35 = 35$

     $x = 0.35$ ml

     16 $\overline{m}$:1 ml::x $\overline{m}$:0.35 ml   PROOF: $16 \times 0.35 = 5.6$

     $x = 16 \times 0.35 = 5.6$ $1 \times 5.6 = 5.6$

     $x = 5.6$ $\overline{m}$

9. **Know**   **Want**

     100 U:1 ml::25 U:x ml   PROOF: $1 \times 25 = 25$

     $100x = 25$ $100 \times 0.25 = 25$

     $x = 0.25$ ml

10. Withdraw insulin to the 30 U calibration. Check order and amount with another nurse.

CHAPTER 7

Insulin Test   (p. 80)

---

1. $x = 0.65$ ml with a tuberculin syringe

2. $x = 0.04$ ml with a tuberculin syringe

3. a. Give 0.16 ml regular insulin with a TB syringe.

     b. Give 0.3 ml NPH insulin with a TB syringe. Check literature to determine if the two can be combined in same syringe.

4. $x = 0.18$ ml with a tuberculin syringe

5. Give 0.16 ml Humulin lente insulin with a tuberculin syringe.

Heparin

☐ **8A**   (p. 82)

1. **Have**   **Want**

   10,~~000~~ U:1 ml::7,~~000~~ U:x ml

   $10x = 7$

   $x = 0.7$ ml

   PROOF: $1 \times 7000 = 7000$

   $10,000 \times 0.7 = 7000$

2. **Have**   **Want**

   20,~~000~~ U:1 ml::15,~~000~~ U:x ml

   $20x = 15$

   $x = 0.75$ ml

   PROOF: $1 \times 15,000 = 15,000$

   $20,000 \times 0.75 = 15,000$

3. **Have**   **Want**

   20,0~~00~~ U:1 ml::25~~00~~ U:x ml

   $200x = 25$

   $x = 0.125 = 0.13$ ml

   PROOF: $200 \times 0.125 = 25$

   $1 \times 25 = 25$

4. **Have**   **Want**

   20,~~000~~ U:1 ml::17,~~000~~ U:x ml $\Big\}$ use the 20,000 U/ml strength

   $20x = 17$

   $x = 0.85$ ml

   PROOF: $1 \times 17 = 17$

   $20 \times 0.85 = 17$

5. **Have**   **Want**

   10,0~~00~~ U:1 ml::75~~00~~ U:x ml

   $100x = 1 \times 75 = 75$

   $100x = 75$

   $x = 0.75$ ml

   PROOF: $1 \times 75 = 75$

   $100 \times 0.75 = 75$

CHAPTER 8

Heparin Test   (p. 83)

1. 0.8 ml
2. 25 U
3. 0.2 ml using the 10,000 U/ml strength
4. 0.35 ml using the 20,000 U/ml strength
5. 0.6 ml

Children's dosages

☐ **9A** (p. 92)

1. a. 14 lb = approximately 7 kg

This is a one-step problem.

Step 1: 2.2 lb:1 kg::14 lb:x kg

$2.2x = 14$

$x = 6.36$ kg

PROOF: $1 \times 14 = 14$

$2.2 \times 6.36 = 13.99$ or 14

b. 12 lb, 2 oz = approximately 6 kg

This is a two-step problem.

Step 1: oz to lb

16 oz:1 lb::2 oz:x lb

$16x = 2$

$x = \frac{1}{8}$ or 0.12 lb   Total weight: 12.12 lb

PROOF: $16 \times 0.12 = 1.92$

$1 \times 2 = 2$

Step 2: lb to kg

2.2 lb:1 kg::12.12:x kg

$2.2x = 12.12$

$x = 5.5$ kg

PROOF: $1 \times 12.12 = 12.12$

$5.5 \times 2.2 = 12.1$

c. 10 lb = approximately 5 kg

This is a one-step problem.

Step 1: 2.2 lb:1 kg::10 lb:x kg

$2.2x = 10$

$x = 4.54$ kg

PROOF: $1 \times 10 = 10$

$2.2 \times 4.54 = 9.988$

d. 7 lb, 6 oz = approximately 3.5 kg

Step 1: oz to lb

16 oz:1 lb::6 oz:x lb

$16x = 6$

$x = 0.37$ lb   Total weight: 7.37 lb

PROOF: $1 \times 6 = 6$

$16 \times 0.37 = 5.92$ or 6

Step 2: lb to kg

Know	Want to know

2.2 lb:1 kg::7.37 lb:x kg

$2.2x = 7.37$

$x = 3.35$ kg

PROOF: $1 \times 7.37 = 7.37$

$2.2 \times 3.35 = 7.37$

e. 15 lb, 8 oz = approximately 7.5 kg
   Step 1: oz to lb

   Know   **Want to know**
   16 oz:1 lb::8 oz:x lb   PROOF: $16 \times .5 = 8$
   $16x = 8$ $1 \times 8 = 8$
   $x = 0.5$ lb   Total weight: 15.5 lb

   Step 2: lb to kg

   Know   **Want to know**
   2.2 lb:1 kg::15.5 lb:x kg   PROOF: $2.2 \times 7 = 15.4$
   $2.2x = 15.5$ $1 \times 15.5 = 15.5$
   $x = 7.0$ kg

2. a. $150 \times 3 = 450$ mg
   b. $200 \times 4 = 800$ mg
   c. $400 \times 6 = 2400$ mg
   d. $50 \times 3 = 150$ mg
   e. $75 \times 2 = 150$ mg

3. a. **Know**   **Want to know**
   10 mg:1 kg::x mg:5 kg   PROOF: $10 \times 5 = 50$
   $x = 10 \times 5$ or 50 mg $1 \times 50 = 50$

   b.   **Know**   **Want to know**
   Step 1: 5 mg:1 kg::x mg:7.3 kg   PROOF: $5 \times 7.3 = 36.5$
   $x = 5 \times 7.3$ or 36.5 mg $1 \times 36.5 = 36.5$

   Know   **Want to know**
   Step 2: 8 mg:1 kg::x mg:7.3 kg   PROOF: $8 \times 7.3 = 58.4$
   $x = 8 \times 7.3$ or 58.4 mg $1 \times 58.4 = 58.4$
   Answer range is 36.5 to 58.4 mg.

   c. 8 lb = approximately 4 kg
   Step 1: lb to kg

   Know   **Want to know**
   2.2 lb:1 kg::8 lb:x kg   PROOF: $2.2 \times 3.63 = 7.98$
   $2.2x = 8$ $1 \times 8 = 8$
   $x = 3.63$ kg (Estimate was 4 kg.)

   Know   **Want to know**
   Step 2: 6 mg:1 kg::x mg:3.63 kg   PROOF: $1 \times 21.78 = 21.78$
   $x = 21.78$ mg $6 \times 3.63 = 21.78$

Step 3: 8 mg:1 kg::*x* mg:3.63 kg   PROOF: 1 × 29.04 = 29.04

        x = 29.04 mg   8 × 3.63 = 29.04

        Answer range is 21.78 mg to 29.04 mg.

d. 5 lb, 8 oz = approximately 2.5 kg

Know   **Want to know**

Step 1: 16 oz:1 lb::8 oz:*x* lb   PROOF: 16 × 0.5 = 8.0

        16*x* = 8   1 × 8 = 8

        x = 0.5 lb

Know   **Want to know**

Step 2: 2.2 lb:1 kg::5.5 lb:*x* kg   PROOF: 1 × 5.5 = 5.5

        2.2*x* = 5.5   2.2 × 2.5 = 5.5

        x = 2.5 kg (Estimate was 2.5 kg.)

Know   **Want to know**

Step 3: 3 mg:1 kg::*x* mg:2.5 kg   PROOF: 3 × 2.5 = 7.5

        x = 7.5 kg   1 × 7.5 = 7.5

Know   **Want to know**

        6 mg:1 kg::*x* mg:2.5 kg   PROOF: 6 × 2.5 = 15

        x = 15.0 mg   1 × 15 = 15

        Answer range is 7.5 to 15 mg.

e. 4 lb, 6 oz = approximately 2 kg

Step 1: oz to lb

Know   **Want to know**

        16 oz:1 lb::6 oz:*x* lb   PROOF: 16 × 0.37 = 5.92

        16*x* = 6   1 × 6 = 6

        x = 6/16 = 0.37 lb

Know   **Want to know**

Step 2: 2.2 lb:1 kg::4.37 lb:*x* kg   PROOF: 2.2 × 1.98 = 4.35

        2.2*x* = 4.37   4.37 = 4.37

        x = 1.98 kg

Know   **Want to know**

Step 3: 20 mg:1 kg::*x* mg:1.98 kg   PROOF: 20 × 1.98 = 39.6

        x = 20 × 1.98   1 × 39.6 = 39.6

        x = 39.6 mg

	Know	**Want to know**	
	40 mg:1 kg::x mg:1.98 kg		PROOF: $40 \times 1.98 = 79.2$
	$x = 40 \times 1.98$		$1 \times 79.2 = 79.2$
	$x = 79.2$ mg		

Answer range is 39.6 to 79.2 mg

4. a. 0.15 m^2
   b. 0.27 m^2
   c. 0.36 m^2
   d. 0.88 − 0.89 m^2
   e. 1.10 m^2

5. a. 0.62 m^2
   b. 0.28 m^2
   c. 0.82 m^2
   d. 0.25 m^2
   e. 0.2 m^2

☐ **9B**   (p. 92)

1. *mg/kg method*
   weight in kg: 7 lb, 2 oz = approximately 3.5 kg

   Know   **Want to know**

   16 oz:1 lb::2 oz:x lb   PROOF: $1 \times 2 = 2$

   $$\frac{16x}{x} = \frac{2}{16} = \frac{1}{8} = 0.125 \text{ lb}$$ $16 \times 0.25 = 2$

   Know   **Want to know**

   2.2 lb:1 kg::7.125 lb:x kg   PROOF: $2.2 \times 3.23 = 7.106$
   $2.2x = 7.125$ $1 \times 7.125 = 7.125$
   $x = 3.23$ kg baby's weight

   safe ranges:

   Know   **Want to know**

   3 mg:1 kg::x mg:3.23 kg   PROOF: $3 \times 3.23 = 9.69$
   $x = 9.69$ mg low safe dose for 24 hours $1 \times 9.69 = 9.69$

   Know   **Want to know**

   6 mg:1 kg::x mg:3.23 kg   PROOF: $6 \times 3.23 = 19.38$
   $x = 19.38$ mg maximum safe dose for 24 hours $1 \times 19.38 = 19.38$

   Doctor ordered 10 mg × 4 or 40 mg total.
   Safe range is 9.69 mg to 19.38 mg for this baby.
   Unsafe order. Hold and clarify promptly.

2. *BSA method*

$$\frac{0.52}{1.7} \times 60 = 18 \text{ mg safe individual dose for this child}$$

Have   **Want to know**

80 mg:2 ml::18 mg:x ml   PROOF: $80 \times 0.45 = 36$

$80x = 36$ $2 \times 18 = 36$

$x = 0.45$ ml

3. *BSA method*

$$\frac{0.6}{1.7} \times 60 = 21 \text{ mg safe individual dose for this child}$$

Know   **Want to know**

4 mg:1 kg::x mg:13.6 kg   PROOF: $1 \times 54.4 = 54.4$

$x = 4 \times 13.6$ or 54.4 mg/24 hours order $4 \times 13.6 = 54.4$

54.5 mg:3 dose::x mg:1 dose   PROOF: $1 \times 54.5 = 54.5$

$3x = 54.5$ $3 \times 18.1 = 54.3$

$x = 18.1$ mg ordered per dose

21 mg safe individual dose (BSA method)
18.1 mg per dose is ordered for this baby.
Safe order

Have   **Want to know**

10 mg:1 ml::18.1 mg:x ml   PROOF: $10 \times 1.8 = 18$

$10x = 18.1$ $1 \times 18.1 = 18.1$

$x = 1.8$ ml

4. *mg/kg method*
estimated kg = 2.5

Know   **Want to know**

16 oz:1 lb::10 oz:x lb   PROOF: $16 \times 0.62 = 9.9$

$16x = 10$ $1 \times 10 = 10$

$x = 0.62$

Baby weighs 5.62 lb.

Know   **Want to know**

2.2 lb:1 kg::5.62 lb:x kg   PROOF: $2.2 \times 2.55 = 5.61$

$2.2x = 5.62$ $1 \times 5.62 = 5.62$

$x = 2.55$ kg

Baby weighs 2.55 kg.

Know   **Want to know**

50 mg:1 kg::x mg:2.55 kg

$x = 50 \times 2.55$

$x = 127.5$ mg safe 24-hour dosage

PROOF: $50 \times 2.55 = 127.5$

$1 \times 127.5 = 127.5$

24-hour doctor order is 50×3 or 150 mg.
Safe limit for 24 hours (mg/kg method) is 127.5 mg.
Unsafe order. Hold and clarify promptly.

5. *mg/kg method*
   estimated weight = 4.5 kg

Know   **Want to know**

16 oz:1 lb::2 oz:x lb

$16x = 2$

$x = 0.125$ lb   Baby weighs 9.125 lb.

PROOF: $16 \times 0.125 = 2$

$1 \times 2 = 2$

Know   **Want to know**

2.2 lb:1 kg::9.125:x lb

$2.2x = 9.125$

$x = 4.14$ kg

PROOF: $2.2 \times 4.14 = 9.108$

$1 \times 9.125 = 9.125$

Know   **Want to know**

20 mg:1 kg::x mg:4.14 kg

$x = 20 \times 4.14$ or 82.8 mg q.12 h

24-hour order is 40 mg $\times$ 2 or 80 mg.

Safe 24-hour dosage by mg/kg method is 82.8 mg $\times$ 2 or 165.6 mg.

Safe order

PROOF: $20 \times 4.14 = 82.8$

$1 \times 82.8 = 82.8$

Have   **Want to know**

300 mg:1 ml::40 mg:x ml

$300x = 40$

$x = 0.13$ ml

PROOF: $300 \times 0.13 = 39$

$1 \times 40 = 40$

☐ **9C**   (p. 94)

1. *mg/kg method*
   30 lb = approximately 15 kg

Know   **Want to know**

2.2 lb:1 kg::30 lb:x kg

$2.2x = 30$

$x = 13.6$ kg

PROOF: $1 \times 30 = 30$

$2.2 \times 13.6 = 29.92$ or 30

Know   **Want to know**

5 mg:1 kg::x mg:13.6 kg

$x = 13.6 \times 5$ or 68.0 mg

24-hour order $= 30 \times 3 = 90$ mg

Safe 24-hour dose $= 68$ mg

Hold and clarify stat.

PROOF: $5 \times 13.6 = 68$

$1 \times 68 = 68$

2. *mg/kg method*

12 lb, 4 oz $=$ approximately 6 kg

Know   **Want to know**

16 oz:1 lb::4 oz:x lb

$16x = 4$

$x = 0.25$ lb   Baby weighs 12.25 lb.

PROOF: $16 \times 0.25 = 4$

$1 \times 4 = 4$

Know   **Want to know**

2.2 lb:1 kg::12.25:x kg

$2.2x = 12.25$

$x = 5.56$ kg

PROOF: $2.2 \times 5.56 = 12.232$

$1 \times 12.25 = 12.25$

Know   **Want to know**

100 mg:1 kg::x mg:5.56 kg

$x = 556$ mg low safe 24-hour dose

PROOF: $1 \times 556 = 556$

$100 \times 5.56 = 556$

200 mg:1 kg::x mg:5.56 kg

$x = 1112$ mg maximum safe 24-hour dose

PROOF: $1 \times 1112 = 1112$

$200 \times 5.56 = 1112$

Doctor ordered 800 mg for 24 hours.

Safe order.

Know   **Want to know**

125 mg:5 ml::200 mg:x ml

$125x = 1000$

$x = 8$ ml

PROOF: $5 \times 200 = 1000$

$125 \times 8 = 1000$

3. $\dfrac{20 \text{ lb}}{150} \times 8 = \dfrac{16}{15} = 1.06$ ml

4. $\dfrac{30 \text{ lb}}{150} \times 5 = \dfrac{5}{5} = 1$ mg

Have   **Want to know**

10 mg:2 ml::1 mg:x ml

$10x = 2$

$x = 0.2$ ml

PROOF: $2 \times 1 = 2$
$10 \times 0.2 = 2.0$

5. $\dfrac{0.84}{1.7} \times 30 = \dfrac{25.2}{1.7} = 14.8$ mg

10 mg h.s. is a safe dose.

☐ 9D   (p. 95)

1. *mg/kg method*
   estimated weight = 24 kg

   Know   **Want to know**

   2.2 lb:1 kg::48 lb:x kg

   $2.2x = 48$

   $x = 21.81$ kg

PROOF: $2.2 \times 21.81 = 47.9$
$1 \times 48 = 48$

   Know   **Want to know**

   2 mg:1 kg::x mg:21.8 kg

   $x = 43.62$ mg low therapeutic dose

PROOF: $2 \times 21.81 = 43.6$
$1 \times 43.6 = 43.6$

   Know   **Want to know**

   6 mg:1 kg::x mg:21.81 kg

   $x = 130.8$ mg safe limit

   Safe range is 43.6 to 130.8 mg.

   120 mg ordered. Save dose. Give.

PROOF: $6 \times 21.81 = 130.8$
$1 \times 130.8 = 130.8$

2. *mg/kg method*
   estimated weight = 10 kg

   Know   **Want to know**

   16 oz:1 lb::8 oz:x lb

   $16x = 8$

   $x = 0.5$ lb

   Baby weighs 20.5 lb.

PROOF: $16 \times 0.5 = 8$
$1 \times 8 = 8$

   Know   **Want to know**

   2.2 lb:1 kg::20.5 lb:x kg

   $2.2x = 20.5$

   $x = 9.31$ kg

   Baby weighs 9.31 kg.

PROOF: $2.2 \times 9.31 = 20.48$
$1 \times 20.5 = 20.5$

Know   Want to know

1 mg:1 kg::x:9.31 kg

x = 9.31 mg

PROOF: $1 \times 9.31 = 9.31$

$1 \times 9.31 = 9.31$

Know   Want to know

2.2 mg:1 kg::x mg:9.31 kg

x = 20.48 mg

Safe range is 9.31 mg to 20.48 mg.

15 mg ordered. Safe order.

PROOF: $2.2 \times 9.31 = 20.48$

$1 \times 20.48 = 20.48$

Have   Want to know

25 mg:1 ml::15 mg:x ml

$25x = 15$

x = 0.6 ml meperidine

PROOF: $25 \times 0.6 = 15.0$

$1 \times 15 = 15$

3. *BSA method*

   BSA for child of normal height for weight is 0.60 m².

   Know   Want to know

   40:1 m²::x mg:0.6 m²

   x = 24.0 mg safe dose for this child

   20 mg ordered. Safe order. Give 20 mg.

   PROOF: $40 \times 0.6 = 24.0$

   $1 \times 24 = 24$

4. *Clark's rule*

$$\frac{3\cancel{0}}{15\cancel{0}} \times 50 = \frac{1}{5} \times 50 = 10 \text{ mg}$$

$$\frac{30}{150} \times 75 = \frac{1}{5} \times 75 = 15 \text{ mg}$$

   Safe range is 10 mg to 15 mg for this child.

   Dose ordered is 25 mg. High.

   Hold and clarify stat. Document.

5. *mg/kg method*

   Estimated kg is 17.5

   Know   Want to know

   2.2 lb:1 kg::35 lb:x kg

   $2.2x = 35$

   x = 15.9 kg

   PROOF: $2.2 \times 15.9 = 34.9$

   $1 \times 35 = 35$

   Know   Want to know

   15 µg:1 kg::x µg:15.9 kg

   x = 15 × 15.9 = 238.5 µg/day safe limit for this child

   PROOF: $15 \times 15.9 = 238.5$

   $1 \times 238.5 = 238.5$

Know	Want to know

1000 μg:1 mg::x μg:0.20 mg   PROOF: $1000 \times 0.20 = 200$

$x = 1000 \times 0.2 = 200$ μg (doctor order) $1 \times 200 = 200$

Safe order. Does not exceed recommended limit.

Have	Want

0.5 mg:1 ml::0.20 mg:x ml   PROOF: $0.5 \times 0.4 = 0.2$

$0.5x = 0.20$ $1 \times 0.20 = 0.2$

$x = 0.4$ ml

Give 0.4 ml.

CHAPTER 9

Children's Dosages Test (p. 96)

1. Safe range is 204.5 to 409 mg daily.
   Safe order; withdraw 4 ml.

2. Safe dosage range is 736 mg to 1472 mg. Withdraw 1 ml from vial for 250 mg per dose.

3. Safe dosage is 22.72 mg. Order is safe at 20 mg. Give 2 ml p.o. stat.

4. 360,000 U. Give 1.2 ml IM.

5. 300,000 U. Give 1 ml IM.

6. 267 mg. Give 3½ tab.

7. 500 mg. Give 10 ml or 2 tsp.

8. Measure 3.75 ml. Measure one full dropper with 2.5 ml and then measure to 1.25 ml calibration on the dropper again to complete the dose.

9. Each teaspoon will contain 250 mg.

10. 54 mg

Basic intravenous calculations

☐ **10A** (p. 102)

KNOW: **1** $\dfrac{TV^*}{TT} = ml/hr$

2 $\dfrac{D^*}{M} \times V = gtt/min$

1. *Step 1:* $\dfrac{TV}{TT} = \dfrac{1000}{8} = 125$ ml/hr

   Step 2: $\dfrac{10}{60} \times \dfrac{125 \ ml}{1} = \dfrac{1}{6} \times \dfrac{125}{1} = \dfrac{125}{6} = 20.8 = 21$ gtt/min

2. *Step 2:* $\dfrac{12}{60} \times \dfrac{200}{1} = \dfrac{1}{5} \times \dfrac{200}{1} = \dfrac{200}{5} = 40$ gtt/min

3. *Step 2:* $\dfrac{10}{30} \times \dfrac{100}{1} = \dfrac{1}{3} \times \dfrac{100}{1} = \dfrac{100}{3} = 33.3$ or 33 gtt/min

4. *Step 1:* $\dfrac{1500}{12} = 125$ ml/hr

   Step 2: $\dfrac{15}{60} \times \dfrac{125}{1} = \dfrac{1}{4} \times \dfrac{125}{1} = 31.2$ or 31 gtt/min

5. *Step 2:* $\dfrac{60}{60} \times \dfrac{50}{1} = \dfrac{1}{1} \times \dfrac{50}{1} = \dfrac{50}{1} = 50$ gtt/min

6. *Step 1:* $\dfrac{1500}{8} = 188$ ml/hr

   Step 2: a. $\dfrac{10}{60} \times \dfrac{188}{1} = \dfrac{1}{6} \times \dfrac{188}{1} = \dfrac{188}{6} = 31.2$ or 31 gtt/min

   b. $\dfrac{15}{60} \times \dfrac{188}{1} = \dfrac{2820}{60} = 47$ gtt/min

---

*Always reduce fraction before multiplying.

7. *Step 2:* $\dfrac{10}{45} \times \dfrac{75}{1} = \dfrac{750}{45} = 16.6$ or 17 gtt/min

8. *Step 2:* $\dfrac{\overset{2}{\cancel{60}}}{\underset{3}{\cancel{90}}} \times 250 = \dfrac{2}{3} \times \dfrac{250}{1} = \dfrac{500}{3} = 166$ gtt/min

9. *Step 2:* $\dfrac{\overset{3}{\cancel{15}}}{\underset{8}{\cancel{40}}} \times 150 = \dfrac{3}{8} \times \dfrac{150}{1} = \dfrac{450}{8} = 56$ gtt/min

10. *Step 2:* $\dfrac{\overset{1}{\cancel{20}}}{\underset{3}{\cancel{60}}} \times 150 = \dfrac{1}{3} \times \dfrac{150}{1} = \dfrac{150}{3} = 50$ gtt/min

☐ **10B**   (p. 104)

REMEMBER: $\dfrac{\text{Total volume}}{\text{Total time}} = \text{ml/hr}$

$\dfrac{\text{Drop factor}}{\text{Time (min)}} \times \text{V/hr} = \text{gtt/min}$

1. *Step 1:* $\dfrac{\text{TV}}{\text{TT}} = \dfrac{2000}{24} = 83.3$ ml/hr

2. *Step 1:* $\dfrac{\text{TV}}{\text{TT}} = \dfrac{1500}{8} = 187.5 = 188$ ml/hr

   Step 2: $\dfrac{15}{60} \times \dfrac{188}{1} = \dfrac{\overset{1}{\cancel{15}}}{\underset{4}{\cancel{60}}} \times \dfrac{188}{1} = 47$ gtt/min

3. *Step 1:* $\dfrac{\text{TV}}{\text{TT}} = \dfrac{3000}{24} = 125$ ml/hr

   Step 2: $\dfrac{60}{60} \times \dfrac{125}{1} = 1 \times 125 = 125$ gtt/min

4. *Step 1:* $\dfrac{TV}{TT} = \dfrac{500}{4} = 125$ ml/hr

Step 2: $\dfrac{\overset{1}{\cancel{15}}}{\underset{4}{\cancel{60}}} \times \dfrac{125}{1} = \dfrac{125}{4} = 31.2 = 31$ gtt/min

5. *Step 1:* $\dfrac{TV}{TT} = \dfrac{1000}{12} = 83.3 = 83$ ml/hr

Step 2: $\dfrac{\overset{1}{\cancel{60}}}{\underset{1}{\cancel{60}}} \times \dfrac{83}{1} = \dfrac{83}{1} = 83$ gtt/min

6. Start with step 2 because we already know how many ml per 30 minutes.

$\dfrac{12}{\underset{3}{\cancel{30}}} \times \dfrac{\overset{10}{\cancel{100}}}{1} = \dfrac{120}{3} = 40$ gtt/min

7. *Step 1:* $\dfrac{TV}{TT} = \dfrac{2000}{24} = 83.3 = 83$ ml/hr

Step 2: $\dfrac{15}{60} \times \dfrac{83}{1} = \dfrac{\overset{1}{\cancel{15}}}{\underset{4}{\cancel{60}}} \times \dfrac{83}{1} = \dfrac{83}{4} = 20.75 = 21$ gtt/min

8. *Step 1:* $\dfrac{TV}{TT} = \dfrac{250}{10} = 25$ ml/hr

Step 2: $\dfrac{\overset{1}{\cancel{60}}}{\underset{1}{\cancel{60}}} \times \dfrac{25}{1} = 25$ gtt/min

9. *Step 1:* $\dfrac{TV}{TT} = \dfrac{1500}{12} = 125$ ml/hr

Step 2: $\dfrac{\overset{1}{\cancel{15}}}{\underset{4}{\cancel{60}}} \times \dfrac{125}{1} = \dfrac{125}{4} = 31$ gtt/min

10. MEMORIZE: $\dfrac{TV}{TT} = \text{ml/hr}$

$$\dfrac{\text{Drop factor}}{\text{Time (min)}} \times \text{V/hr} = \text{gtt/min} \quad \text{or} \quad \dfrac{D}{M} \times V = \text{gtt/min}$$

□ **10C** (p. 106)

REMEMBER: *Step 1:* $\dfrac{TV}{TT} = \text{ml/hr}$

$\qquad\qquad$ *Step 2:* $\dfrac{D}{M} \times V = \text{gtt/min}$

1. *Step 2:* $\dfrac{1\cancel{0}}{6\cancel{0}} \times 100 = \dfrac{100}{6} = 16.6 = 17 \text{ gtt/min}$

2. *Step 1:* $\dfrac{TV}{TT} = \dfrac{1000}{6} = 166.6 = 167 \text{ ml/hr}$

$\qquad$ *Step 2:* $\dfrac{15}{60} \times \dfrac{167}{1} = \dfrac{\overset{1}{\cancel{15}}}{\underset{4}{\cancel{60}}} \times \dfrac{167}{1} = \dfrac{167}{4} = 41.75 = 42 \text{ gtt/min}$

3. *Step 2:* $\dfrac{10}{30} \times \dfrac{50}{1} = \dfrac{1\cancel{0}}{3\cancel{0}} \times \dfrac{50}{1} = \dfrac{50}{3} = 16.6 = 17 \text{ gtt/min}$

4. *Step 2:* $\dfrac{60}{60} \times \dfrac{100}{1} = \dfrac{\overset{1}{\cancel{60}}}{\underset{1}{\cancel{60}}} \times \dfrac{100}{1} = 100 \text{ gtt/min}$

5. *Step 1:* $\dfrac{TV}{TT} = \dfrac{2000}{12} = 166.6 = 167 \text{ ml/hr}$

$\qquad$ *Step 2:* $\dfrac{60}{60} \times \dfrac{167}{1} = \dfrac{\overset{1}{\cancel{60}}}{\underset{1}{\cancel{60}}} \times \dfrac{167}{1} = 167 \text{ gtt/min}$

6. *Step 2:* $\dfrac{12}{30} \times \dfrac{100}{1} = \dfrac{12}{3\cancel{0}} \times \dfrac{10\cancel{0}}{1} = \dfrac{120}{3} = 40 \text{ gtt/min}$

7. *Step 1:* $\dfrac{\text{TV}}{\text{TT}} = \dfrac{1500}{24} = 62.5 = 63$ ml/hr

   Step 2: $\dfrac{10}{60} \times \dfrac{63}{1} = \dfrac{1\cancel{0}}{6\cancel{0}} \times \dfrac{63}{1} = \dfrac{63}{6} \times 10.5 = 11$ gtt/min

8. *Step 1:* $\dfrac{\text{TV}}{\text{TT}} = \dfrac{500}{8} = 62.5 = 63$ ml/hr

   Step 2: $\dfrac{60}{60} \times \dfrac{63}{1} = \dfrac{\overset{1}{\cancel{60}}}{\underset{1}{\cancel{60}}} \times \dfrac{63}{1} = 63$ gtt/min

9. *Step 2:* $\dfrac{15}{60} \times 75 = \dfrac{1}{4} \times \dfrac{75}{1} = \dfrac{75}{4} = 19$ gtt/min

10. *Step 2:* $\dfrac{20}{60} \times 85 = \dfrac{1}{3} \times \dfrac{85}{1} = \dfrac{85}{3} = 28.3 = 28$ gtt/min

☐ **10D**   (p. 108)

1. $\dfrac{15}{60} \times \dfrac{100}{1} = \dfrac{1}{4} \times \dfrac{100}{1} = \dfrac{100}{4} = 25$ gtt/min

2. $\dfrac{15}{20} \times \dfrac{50}{1} = \dfrac{\overset{3}{\cancel{15}}}{\underset{4}{\cancel{20}}} \times \dfrac{50}{1} = \dfrac{150}{4} = 37.5$ or 38 gtt/min

3. $\dfrac{60}{30} \times \dfrac{50}{1} = \dfrac{\overset{2}{\cancel{60}}}{\underset{1}{\cancel{30}}} \times \dfrac{50}{1} = 100$ gtt/min

4. $\dfrac{12}{60} \times \dfrac{100}{1} = \dfrac{\overset{1}{\cancel{12}}}{\underset{5}{\cancel{60}}} \times \dfrac{100}{1} = \dfrac{100}{5} = 20$ gtt/min

5.   **Know**   **Want to know**

   Step 1: 20 gtt:1 ml::x gtt:250 ml

   $x = 20 \times 250 = 5000$

   $x = 5000$ gtt in 250 ml

Step 2: 60 gtt:1 minute::5000 gtt:x minutes

$$60x = 5000 = \frac{5000}{60}$$

$x = 83.3$ minutes $= 1$ hour, 23 minutes

6.   **Know**   **Want to know**

Step 1: 15 gtt:1 ml::x gtt:2000 ml

$x = 15 \times 2000 = 30,000$

$x = 30,000$ gtt in 2000 ml

               Know   **Want to know**

Step 2: 40 gtt:1 minute::30,000 gtt:x minutes

$$40x = 30,000 = \frac{30,00\!\!\!/}{4\!\!\!/} = 750$$

$x = 750$ minutes $= 12\frac{1}{2}$ hours to infuse

7. $\dfrac{\overset{3}{\cancel{60}}}{\underset{2}{\cancel{40}}} \times 150 = \dfrac{450}{2} = 225$ gtt/min is the fastest rate

$\dfrac{\cancel{60}}{\cancel{60}} \times 150 = 150$ gtt/min is the slowest rate

8.   **Know**   **Want to know**

Step 1: 15 gtt:1 ml::x gtt:1000 ml

$x = 15 \times 1000 = 15,000$

$x = 15,000$ gtt in 1000 ml

               Know   **Want to know**

Step 2: 40 gtt:1 minute::15,000 gtt:x minutes

$40x = 15,000$

$x = 375$ minutes $= 6$ hours, 15 minutes to infuse

9. $\dfrac{\overset{2}{\cancel{60}}}{\underset{1}{\cancel{30}}} \times 100 = 200$ gtt/min

10.

	Know	Want to know

Step 1: 60 gtt:1 ml::x gtt:200 ml

$x = 60 \times 200 = 12{,}000$

$x = 12{,}000$ gtt in 200 ml

	Know	Want to know

Step 2: 50 gtt:1 minute::12,000 gtt:x minutes

$50x = 12{,}000$

$x = 240$ minutes = 4 hours

☐ **10E** (p. 109)

1. $\dfrac{\overset{1}{\cancel{20}}}{\underset{3}{\cancel{60}}} \times 40 = \dfrac{40}{3} = 13$ gtt/min

2. $\dfrac{\overset{1}{\cancel{15}}}{\underset{4}{\cancel{60}}} \times 80 = \dfrac{80}{4} = 20$ gtt/min

Know **Want to know**

80 ml:1 hr::x ml:24 hr

$x = 80 \times 24 = 1920$

$x = 1920$ ml in 24 hr

3. $\dfrac{60}{60} \times 125 = 125$ gtt/min and 125 ml/hr

4. $\dfrac{3000}{24} = 125$ ml/hr = 125 gtt/min

5. $\dfrac{2000}{24} = 83.3 = 83$ ml/hr

$\dfrac{\overset{1}{\cancel{20}}}{\underset{3}{\cancel{60}}} \times 83 = \dfrac{83}{3} = 27.6 = 28$ gtt/min

1. **Know**   **Want to know**

   125 ml:1 hour::100 ml:x hours

   125 x = 1000

   x = 8 hours

   PROOF: 125 × 8 = 1000

   1 × 1000 = 1000

   Know   **Want to know**

   8 hours:10 U::1 hour:x U

   8x = 10 × 1 = 10

   x = 1.25 U/hour

   PROOF: 1 × 10 = 10

   8 × 1.25 = 10

2. **Know**   **Want to know**

   150 ml:1 hour::1000 ml:x hours

   150x = 1000

   x = 6.6 hours = 6 hours, 36 minutes

   PROOF: 1 × 1000 = 1000

   6.6 × 150 = 990

   Know   **Want to know**

   6.6 hours:20 U::1 hour:x U

   $6.6x = 20 \times 1 = \dfrac{20}{6.6} = 3$

   x = 3 U/hr

   PROOF: 20 × 1 = 20

   6.6 × 3 = 19.8

3. **Know**   **Want to know**

   40 g:1000 ml::2 g:x ml

   40x = 1000 × 2 = 2000

   40x = 2000

   x = 50 ml/hr = 2 g MgSO$_4$ = 50 gtt/min

   50 ml:1 hour::1000 ml:x hours

   50x = 1000

   x = 20 hours to infuse

   PROOF: 40 × 50 = 2000

   2 × 1000 = 2000

   PROOF: 1 × 1000 = 1000

   50 × 20 = 1000

4. **Know**   **Want to know**

   20 g:1000 ml::x g:25 ml

   1000x = 20 × 25 = 500

   1000x = 500

   x = 0.5 g/hr = 500 mg/hr

   $\dfrac{60}{60} \times 25$ ml/hr = 25 gtt/min

   PROOF: 20 × 25 = 500

   0.5 × 1000 = 500

   Know   **Want to know**

   25 ml:1 hour::1000 ml:x hours

   25x = 1000

   x = 40 hours to infuse

   PROOF: 1 × 1000 = 1000

   25 × 40 = 1000

5. **Know**   **Want to know**

1000 ml:40 g::x ml:3 g

$40x = 3 \times 1000 = 3000$

$40x = 3000$

$x = 75$ ml/hr = 75 gtt/min

PROOF: $40 \times 75 = 3000$

$3 \times 1000 = 3000$

Know   **Want to know**

75 ml:1 hour::1000 ml:x hours

$75x = 1000$

$x = 13.3$ hours = 13 hours, 18 minutes to infuse

PROOF: $1 \times 1000 = 1000$

$75 \times 13.3 = 997.5$

☐ **10G**   (p. 112)

1. **Know**   **Want to know**

20,000 U:1000 ml::1000 U:x ml

$20x = 1000 \times 1 = 1000$

$20x = 1000$

$x = 50$ ml/hr = 1000 U heparin

$\dfrac{60}{60} \times 50 = 50$ gtt/min

PROOF: $20{,}000 \times 50 = 1{,}000{,}000$

$1000 \times 1000 = 1{,}000{,}000$

2. $\dfrac{1000}{12} = 83.3 = 83$ ml/hr

$\dfrac{60}{60} \times 83 = 83$ gtt/min

Know   **Want to know**

20,000 U:12 hours::x U:1 hour

$12x = 20{,}000$

$x = 1666$ U/hr

PROOF: $20{,}000 \times 1 = 20{,}000$

$12 \times 1666 = 19{,}992$

3. **Know**   **Want to know**

20000 U:1000 ml::1500 U:x ml

$200x = 15000$

$x = 75$ ml/hr = 1500 U heparin

$\dfrac{60}{60} \times 75 = 75$ gtt/min

PROOF: $200 \times 75 = 15{,}000$

$1000 \times 15 = 15{,}000$

Know   **Want to know**

75 ml:1 hour::1000 ml:x hours

$75x = 1000$

$x = 13.3$ hours = 13 hours, 18 minutes to infuse

PROOF: $1 \times 1000 = 1000$

$75 \times 13.3 = 997.5$

4. **Know**   **Want to know**

10,000 U:15 hours::x U:1 hour

$15x = 1 \times 10,000 = 10,000$

$x = 666$ U/hr

$$\frac{1000}{15} = 66.6 = 67 \text{ ml/hr} = 67 \text{ gtt/min}$$

PROOF: $15 \times 666 = 9990$

$10,000 \times 1 = 10,000$

5. **Know**   **Want to know**

10,0̸0̸0̸ U:500 ml::12̸0̸0̸ U:x ml

$100x = 500 \times 12 = 6000$

$10̸0̸x = 60̸0̸0̸$

$x = 60$ ml/hr $= 1200$ U heparin

$$\frac{60}{60} \times 60 = 60 \text{ gtt/min}$$

PROOF: $500 \times 12 = 6000$

$100 \times 60 = 6000$

6. **Know**   **Want to know**

500 ml:250 U::x ml:10 U

$250x = 500 \times 10 = 5000$

$25̸0̸x = 500̸0̸$

$x = 20$ ml/hr $= 10$ U

PROOF: $500 \times 10 = 5000$

$250 \times 20 = 5000$

Know   **Want to know**

20 ml:1 hour::500 ml:x hours

$20x = 500$

$x = 25$ hours to infuse

$$\frac{60}{60} \times 20 = 20 \text{ gtt/min}$$

PROOF: $1 \times 500 = 500$

$20 \times 25 = 500$

7. **Know**   **Want to know**

250 ml:100 U::x ml:6 U

$100x = 250 \times 6 = 1500$

$x = 15$ ml/hr $= 15$ gtt/min to deliver 6 U insulin

PROOF: $250 \times 6 = 1500$

$6 \times 250 = 1500$

Know   **Want to know**

15 ml:1 hour::250 ml:x hours

$15x = 250$

$x = 16.6$ hours

PROOF: $1 \times 250 = 250$

$15 \times 16.6 = 249$

8. **Know**   **Want to know**

100 U:250 ml::8 U:x ml

$100x = 250 \times 8 = 2000$

$1\cancel{0}\cancel{0}x = 200\cancel{0}$

$x = 20$ ml/hr = 8 U insulin

$\dfrac{60}{60} \times 20 = 20$ gtt/min

PROOF: $250 \times 8 = 2000$

$100 \times 20 = 2000$

Know   **Want to know**

20 ml:1 hour::250 ml:x hours

$20x = 250$

$x = 12.5$ hours to infuse

PROOF: $20 \times 12.5 = 250$

$1 \times 250 = 250$

9. **Know**   **Want to know**

200 ml:100 U::x ml:7 U

$100x = 200 \times 7 = 1400$

$1\cancel{0}\cancel{0}x = 140\cancel{0}$

$x = 14$ ml/hr = 14 gtt/min

PROOF: $200 \times 7 = 1400$

$100 \times 14 = 1400$

Know   **Want to know**

14 ml:1 hour::200 ml:x hours

$14x = 200$

$x = 14.2$ hours to infuse

PROOF: $14 \times 14.2 = 198.8$

$1 \times 200 = 200$

10. **Know**   **Want to know**

500 ml:100 U::x ml:9 U

$100x = 500 \times 9 = 4500$

$1\cancel{0}\cancel{0}x = 450\cancel{0}$

$x = 45$ ml/hr = 45 gtt/min to deliver 9 U insulin

PROOF: $500 \times 9 = 4500$

$100 \times 45 = 4500$

Know   **Want to know**

45 ml:1 hour::500 ml:x hours

$45x = 500$

$x = 11.1$ hours to infuse

PROOF: $45 \times 11.1 = 499.5$

$1 \times 500 = 500$

Basic Intravenous Calculations Test   (p. 113)

1. 125ml/hr
   31 gtt/min
   (Step 1)
2. 17 gtt/min
   (Step 2)
3. 83 ml/hr
   17 gtt/min
   (Step 1)
4. 150 ml/hr
   150 gtt/min
   (Step 1)

5. 83 ml/hr
   14 gtt/min
   (Step 1)
6. 125 ml/hr
   31 gtt/min
   (Step 1)
7. 125 ml/hr
   125 gtt/min
   (Step 1)

8. 83 ml/hr
   18 gtt/min
   (Step 1)
9. 83 ml/hr
   83 gtt/min
   (Step 1)
10. 166 gtt/min
    (Step 2)

CHAPTER 11

Intravenous titrations

☐ 11A   (p. 118)

Convert lb to kg.

1. **Know   Want to know**
   1 kg:2.2 lb::x kg:135 lb
   $2.2x = 135$
   $x = 61.3$ kg

   PROOF: $2.2 \times 61.3 = 135$
   $1 \times 135 = 135$

2. **Know   Want to know**
   1 kg:2.2 lb::x kg:205 lb
   $2.2x = 205$
   $x = 93.1$ kg

   PROOF: $2.2 \times 93.1 = 205$
   $1 \times 205 = 205$

3. **Know   Want to know**
   1 kg:2.2 lb::x kg:98 lb
   $2.2x = 98$
   $x = 44.5$ kg

   PROOF: $2.2 \times 44.5 = 98$
   $1 \times 98 = 98$

4. **Know   Want to know**
   1 kg:2.2 lb::x kg:176 lb
   $2.2x = 176$
   $x = 80$ kg

   PROOF: $2.2 \times 80 = 176$
   $1 \times 176 = 176$

5. **Know**   **Want to know**

    1 kg:2.2 lb::x kg:159 lb

    2.2x = 159

    x = 72.2 kg

PROOF: 2.2 × 72.2 = 159

1 × 159 = 159

Calculate µg/kg/min and mg/kg/min.

6. weight = 61.3 kg

    Know   **Want to know**

    15 µg:1 kg::x µg:61.3 kg

    x = 15 × 61.3 = 919

    x = 919 µg/min for weight of 61.3 kg

PROOF: 15 × 61.3 = 919

1 × 919 = 919

7. weight = 93.1 kg

    Know   **Want to know**

    10 µg:1 kg::x µg:93.1 kg

    x = 10 × 93.1 = 931

    x = 931 µg/min for weight of 93.1 kg

PROOF: 10 × 93.1 = 931

1 × 931 = 931

8. weight = 44.5 kg

    Know   **Want to know**

    7 µg:1 kg::x µg:44.5 kg

    x = 7 × 44.5 = 311

    x = 311 µg/min for weight of 44.5 kg

PROOF: 7 × 44.5 = 311

1 × 311 = 311

9. weight = 80 kg

    Know   **Want to know**

    0.003 mg:1 kg::x mg:80 kg

    x = 0.003 × 80 = 0.24

    x = 0.24 mg/min for weight of 80 kg

PROOF: 0.003 × 80 = 0.24

1 × 0.24 = 0.24

10. weight = 72.2 kg

    Know   **Want to know**

    0.006 mg:1 kg::x mg:72.2 kg

    x = 0.006 × 72.2 = 0.433

    x = 0.433 mg/min for weight of 72.2 kg

PROOF: 0.006 × 72.2 = 0.433

1 × 0.433 = 0.433

Calculate minutes/infusion time.

11. **Know   Want to know**

919 μg:1 minute::50,000 μg: x minutes   PROOF: $1 \times 50,000 = 50,000$
919x = 50,000 $919 \times 54 = 49,626$
x = 54 minutes to infuse

12. **Know   Want to know**

931 μg:1 minute::50,000 μg:x minutes   PROOF: $931 \times 54 = 50,274$
931x = 50,000 $1 \times 50,000 = 50,000$
x = 54 minutes to infuse

13. **Know   Want to know**

1 mg:1000 μg:x mg:311 μg   PROOF: $1 \times 311 = 311$
1000x = 311 $1000 \times 0.311 = 311$
x = 0.311 mg

Know   Want to know

0.311 mg:1 minute::20 mg: x minutes   PROOF: $0.311 \times 64 = 19.9$
0.311x = 20 $1 \times 20 = 20$
x = 64 minutes to infuse

14. **Know   Want to know**

0.24 mg:1 minute::20 mg: x minutes   PROOF: $1 \times 20 = 20$
0.24x = 20 $0.24 \times 83 = 19.9$
x = 83 minutes to infuse

15. **Know   Want to know**

1 mg:1000 μg::0.006 mg: x μg   PROOF: $1 \times 6 = 6$
x = 1000 × 0.006 = 6 $1000 \times 0.006 = 6$
x = 6 μg

Know   Want to know

6 μg:1 minute::500 μg:x minutes   PROOF: $6 \times 83 = 498$
6x = 500 $1 \times 500 = 500$
x = 83 minutes to infuse

☐ **11B**   (p. 120)

1. Dobutamine
   Step 1: lb to kg

   Know   Want to know

   1 kg:2.2 lb:: x kg:155 lb   PROOF: $1 \times 155 = 155$
   2.2x = 155 $2.2 \times 70.4 = 154.8$
   x = 70.4 kg

Step 2: μg to mg

Know   **Want to know**

1 mg:1000 μg::*x* mg:10 μg   PROOF: 1 × 10 = 10
1000*x* = 1 × 10 = 10   1000 × 0.01 = 10
x = 0.01 mg

Step 3: mg/kg/min

Know   **Want to know**

0.01 mg:1 kg::*x* mg:70.4 kg   PROOF: 0.01 × 70.4 = 0.704
x = 0.01 × 70.4 = 0.704   1 × 0.704 = 0.704
x = 0.704 mg/min for 70.4 kg weight

Step 4: minutes to deliver 200 mg

Know   **Want to know**

0.704 mg:1 minute::200 mg:*x* minutes   PROOF: 1 × 200 = 200
0.704*x* = 200   0.704 × 284 = 199
x = 284 minutes ÷ 60 = 4 hours, 44 minutes

Step 5: medication amount

Know   **Want to know**

250 mg:20 ml::200 mg:*x* ml   PROOF: 250 × 16 = 4000
250*x* = 20 × 200 = 4000   20 × 200 = 4000
250*x* = 4000
x = 16 ml   Dilute to 50 ml of IV solution.

Step 6: $\dfrac{60}{284} \times 50 = \dfrac{3000}{284} = 10.5 = 11$ gtt/min

The current rate of infusion is 125 ml/hr with a microdrip, which means 125 gtt/min. Therefore, the IV rate must be changed to 11 gtt/min until 50 ml is infused, which will take 4 hours, 44 minutes.

2. Nitroprusside
    Step 1: lb to kg

Know   **Want to know**

1 kg:2.2 1b::*x* kg:165 lb   PROOF: 2.2 × 75 = 165
2.2*x* = 165   1 × 165 = 165
x = 75 kg

Step 2: μg to mg conversion

Know   **Want to know**

1 mg:1000 μg::*x* mg:3 μg   PROOF: 0.003 × 1000 = 3
1000*x* = 3 × 1 = 3   1 × 3 = 3
x = 0.003 mg

Step 3: mg/kg/min

Know **Want to know**

0.003 mg:1 kg::x mg:75 kg

$x = 0.003 \times 75 = 0.225$

$x = 0.225$ mg/min

PROOF: $1 \times 0.225 = 0.225$
$0.003 \times 75 = 0.225$

Step 4: mg/min

Know **Want to know**

0.225 mg:1 minute::50 mg:x minutes

$0.225x = 50$

$x = 222.2$ minutes $\div$ 60 = 3 hours, 42 minutes

PROOF: $1 \times 50 = 50$
$0.225 \times 222.2 = 49.995$

Step 5: gtt/min

$$\dfrac{\overset{20}{\cancel{60}}}{\underset{74}{\cancel{222}}} \times 250 = \dfrac{5000}{74} = 67.5 = 68 \text{ gtt/min}$$

Step 6: The current rate of infusion is 85 ml/hr or 85 gtt/min. The rate for nitroprusside is 68 gtt/min; the rate has to be decreased for 3 hours, 42 minutes.

3. Lidocaine

Step 1: lb to kg

Know **Want to know**

1 kg:2.2 lb::x kg:182 lb

$2.2x = 182$

$x = 82.7$ kg

PROOF: $2.2 \times 82.7 = 181.9$
$1 \times 182 = 182$

Step 2: maximum dose for patient using μg/min

Know **Want to know**

50 μg:1 kg::x μg:82.7 kg

$x = 50 \times 82.7 = 4135$

$x = 4135$ μg/min for patient weighing 82.7 kg

PROOF: $1 \times 4135 = 4135$
$50 \times 82.7 = 4135$

Step 3: convert μg to mg

Know **Want to know**

1 mg:1000 μg::x mg:4135 μg

$1000x = 4135$

$x = 4.135$ mg/min for weight of 82.7 kg

Therefore, 4.0 mg/min order is safe.

PROOF: $1 \times 4135 = 4135$
$1000 \times 4.135 = 4135$

■ 205

Step 4: mg/hr (min) Is this a safe dose for 1 hour?

Know   **Want to know**

4 mg:1 minute::x mg:60 minutes   PROOF: $1 \times 240 = 240$

$x = 4 \times 60 = 240$ $4 \times 60 = 240$

$x = 240$ mg/hr

This is a safe dose. Literature states no more than 300 mg over a 1-hour period.

Step 5: ml/hr

Know   **Want to know**

1 mg:1 ml::240 mg:x ml   PROOF: $1 \times 240 = 240$

$x = 240$ ml/hr = 240 gtt/min (microdrip) $1 \times 240 = 240$

Change existing IV rate from 100 ml/hr to 240 ml/hr.

4. Coly-Mycin M

Know   **Want to know**

Step 1: 1 kg:2.2 lb::x kg:176 lb   PROOF: $1 \times 176 = 176$

$2.2x = 176$ $2.2 \times 80 = 176$

$x = 80$ kg

Step 2: safe dose

Know   **Want to know**

5 mg:1 kg::x mg:80 kg   PROOF: $5 \times 80 = 400$

$x = 80 \times 5 = 400$ $1 \times 400 = 400$

$x = 400$ mg/24 hr = maximum dose

Ordered: 150 mg q.12h. = 300 mg/24 hrs. This is a safe dose.

Know   **Want to know**

Step 3: 1 ml:75 mg::x ml:150 mg   PROOF: $75 \times 2 = 150$

$75x = 150$ $1 \times 150 = 150$

$x = 2$ ml   Further dilute to 100 ml for volutrol infusion.

Step 4: $\dfrac{\overset{3}{\cancel{60}}}{\underset{2}{\cancel{40}}} \times 100 = \dfrac{300}{2} = 150$ gtt/min or $\dfrac{\overset{3}{\cancel{60}}}{\underset{1}{\cancel{20}}} \times 100 = 300$ gtt/min

Use existing IV rate of 150 ml/hr and IV will be infused in 40 minutes.

5. Aldomet

   Step 1: lb/kg

Know	Want to know

   1 kg:2.2 lb::x kg:155 lb

   $2.2x = 155$

   $x = 70.4$ kg

   PROOF: $1 \times 155 = 155$
   $2.2 \times 70.4 = 154.88$

   Step 2: maximum dose

Know	Want to know

   10 mg:1 kg::x mg:70.4 kg

   $x = 70.4 \times 10 = 704$

   $x = 704$ mg q.6h. is the maximum dose

   PROOF: $1 \times 704 = 704$
   $10 \times 70.4 = 704$

   Step 3: convert g to mg

Know	Want to know

   1 g:1000 mg::0.5 g:x mg

   $x = 1000 \times 0.5 = 500$

   $x = 500$ mg q.6h. ordered. Safe dose

   low dose

Know	Want to know

   7 mg:1 kg::x mg:70.4 kg

   $x = 7 \times 70.4 = 492.8$

   $x = 492.8$ mg q.6h.

   500 mg q.6h. is the low dose.

   PROOF: $1 \times 500 = 500$
   $1000 \times 0.5 = 500$

   PROOF: $1 \times 492.8 = 492.8$
   $7 \times 70.4 = 492.8$

   Step 4: $\dfrac{60}{60} \times 200 = 200$ gtt/min   Change rate from 100 gtt/min to 200 gtt/min.

CHAPTER 12

Solutions

☐ **12A**   (p. 126)

1. **Have**   **Want**

   0.9 g:100 ml::x g NaC1:500 ml water

   $100x = 450$

   $x = 4.5$ g salt added to 500 ml water

   PROOF: $0.9 \times 500 = 450$
   $100 \times 4.5 = 450$

   REMEMBER: 1 tsp = 4 to 5 ml or g

2. **Have   Want**

$50:100::x:200$

$100x = 10,000$

$x = 100$ ml 0.45% normal saline

$$\begin{array}{r} 200 \\ -100 \\ \hline \end{array} \text{0.45\% normal saline}$$

Add   100 ml peroxide.

PROOF: $100 \times 100 = 10,000$

$50 \times 200 = 10,000$

3. **Have   Want**

5 ml:100 ml::x ml acetic acid:300 ml water

$100x = 1500$

$x = 15$ ml acetic acid

Pour 15 ml of 5% acetic acid into a container. Then add water to the 300 ml mark.

$$\begin{array}{r} 300 \text{ ml desired} \\ -15 \text{ ml acetic acid} \\ \hline 285 \text{ ml water} \end{array}$$

PROOF: $100 \times 15 = 1500$

$5 \times 300 = 1500$

4. **Have   Want**

10 ml:100 ml::x ml acetic acid:250 ml

$100x = 2500$

$x = 25$ ml acetic acid

Pour 25 ml full-strength acetic acid into container. Then add water to the 250 ml mark.

$$\begin{array}{r} 250 \text{ ml desired} \\ -25 \text{ ml acetic acid} \\ \hline 225 \text{ ml water} \end{array}$$

PROOF: $10 \times 250 = 2500$

$100 \times 25 = 2500$

5. **Have   Want**

0.9 g:100 ml::x g salt:150 ml

$100x = 135$

$x = 1.35 = 1$ ml or g salt

PROOF: $100 \times 1.35 = 135$

$0.9 \times 150 = 135$

Add 1 g of salt to 150 ml of water. Because it is difficult to measure 1 g or ml of salt, just make up a normal saline solution of 500 ml water (1 pt) and add 1 tsp (4 to 5 ml) of salt. Discard any unused portion.

6. **Have**   **Want**

     10 ml:100 ml::x ml acetic acid:200 ml water   PROOF: $100 \times 20 = 2000$

     $100x = 2000$ $10 \times 200 = 2000$

     $x = 20$ ml acetic acid

     Add 20 ml of 10% acetic acid to the container; add water to make 200 ml.

     200 ml desired
     $-$ 20 ml acetic acid
     180 ml water

7. **Have**   **Want**

     0.9 g:100 ml::x g NaCl:1000 ml water   PROOF: $100 \times 9 = 900$

     $100x = 900$ $0.9 \times 1000 = 900$

     $x = 9$ g NaCl or 2 tsp

     Always prepare a 1000 ml solution for an enema.

8. **Have**   **Want**

     0.9 g:100 ml::x g NaCl:500 ml water   PROOF: $100 \times 4.5 = 450$

     $100x = 450$ $0.9 \times 500 = 450$

     $x = 4.5$ g salt = 1 tsp.

     You should have this problem memorized by now. REMEMBER: 1 tsp in 1 pint of water gives 500 ml of normal saline solution.

9. **Have**   **Want**

     1½ ml:100 ml::x ml vinegar:1000 ml   PROOF: $100 \times 15 = 1500$

                                                           $1½ \times 1000 = 1500$

     $100x = \dfrac{3}{2} \times 1000 = 1500$

     $100x = 1500$
     $x = 15$ ml vinegar

     Add 15 ml or 3 tsp of vinegar to the 1 L container. Add 985 ml water to make up 1000 ml of solution.

10. **Have**   **Want**

     40 ml bet.:100 ml sol::x ml Betadine:500 ml normal saline   PROOF: $100 \times 200 = 20,000$

     $100\ x = 40 \times 500 = 20,000$ $40 \times 500 = 20,000$

     $10\cancel{0}x = 20,0\cancel{00}$
     $x = 200$ ml Betadine

         500 ml desired
         $-$ 200 ml full-strength Betadine
   add   300 ml normal saline

Solutions Test   (p. 128)

1. *Pour:*   8 ml Lysol

   Add: <u>3992 ml</u> water
                 4000 ml of a 1:500 solution of Lysol

2. *Pour:*   125 ml Betadine needed

   Add: <u>125 ml</u> 0.45% normal saline
                 250 ml

   This means dissolve gr 30 (or six 5-gr tablets) in 1000 ml of a 1:500 solution.

3. *Pour:*   1.3 ml $KMnO_4$

   Add: <u>998.7 ml</u>
                 1000 ml = 1:750 solution

4. Each tablet of $KMnO_4$ contains 1 gr. Dissolve 10½ tablets of $KMnO_4$ (1 gr each) in 500 ml of water to make 500 ml of 1:750 solution.

5. *Pour:*   90 ml peroxide

   Add: <u>210 ml</u> solution
                 300 ml use 0.9% saline

Comprehensive examination   (p. 129)

1. 2 ml dose and 6 ml per day   8. 125 ml/hr

2. 6 ml   9. 17 gtt/min

3. 2 tab.   10. 1 ml

4. 0.4 ml   11. 1.3 ml

5. 2 ml   12. 1.5 ml

6. 63 ml/hr   13. 0.7 ml

7. 16 gtt/min   14. 2 tab.

15. 0.5 ml

16. 0.24 ml

17. 6 minims

18. 0.25 ml

19. 1.3 ml

20. 0.5 ml

21. 1 tsp

22. 1 suppository

23. 100 ml

24. 15 ml or 3 tsp

25. 2 tab.

26. 121 lb

27. 39.2 mg; hold and clarify

28. 70 to 141 mg; unsafe

29. 40 gtt/min

30. 25 gtt/min

Index

P.98 – IV's

$$\frac{TV}{TV} = ml/hr$$

$$\frac{D}{M} \times V$$